THE
KNOCKOUT
WORKOUT

3 Winning Steps to Improve Your Body and Your Life

MIA ST. JOHN

with Robert Wolff

TRADE PAPER
PRESS

Trade Paper Press
An imprint of Turner Publishing Company
Nashville, Tennessee
www.turnerpublishing.com

Photo credits: pp. 48, 15, 159, Bill Dobbins; pp. 54, 56, 58, 59, 62, 63, 66, 67, 68, 70, 75, 129, Fernando Escovar; pp. 52, 55, 61, 64, 71, 72, 73, 74, 76, 77, 125, 126, 127, 131, 132, 136, 137, 138, 141, 143, 145, 146, 147, 152, 153, 155, 160, 166, 168, 171, 178, 186, 188, Jonathan White

Library of Congress Cataloging-in-Publication Data:

St. John, Mia, date.
  The knockout workout : 3 winning steps to improve your body and your life / Mia St. John.
      p. cm.
  Includes index.
  ISBN 978-0-470-26750-9 (cloth : alk. paper)
  1. Exercise—Popular works. 2. Physical fitness—Popular works. I. Title.
  RA781.S696 2009
  613.7'1—dc22

                                                        2008055888

Printed in the United States of America

10   9   8   7   6   5   4   3   2

In memory of my beloved first trainer,
Art Lovett,
February 4, 1943–June 17, 1997

CONTENTS

PREFACE

Vision without action is a daydream.
Action without vision is a nightmare.
—JAPANESE PROVERB

Before I tell you more about this amazing exercise and diet lifestyle, I think it might surprise you to learn that I once struggled with and overcame an eating disorder. And I'm not alone—far from it. I see so many women who have had (and may *still* have) the same problem. But help has arrived.

The Knockout Workout speaks to any woman who has a love-hate relationship with food and with her body. In my experience, that describes roughly 90 percent of the women in developed countries.

The evolution of this plan dates back to 1996, before I learned the powerful lessons that transformed me into the strong, fit, confident woman I am today. Yet perhaps equally important are the years leading up to 1996: the story of who I am and where I came from.

When I was a child, I had dreams of escaping my dysfunctional family, my insecurities, and myself. My father was a tall, dark, handsome man, with muscular arms bearing tattoos he'd acquired while serving in the navy.

When he was stationed in San Diego, he often crossed the border into Mexico. There he met my mother, while dining at the restaurant where she worked. He practiced his Spanish with her, and because she knew very little English, she did the same with his native language.

They fell in love almost immediately. My mother was beautiful, with long black hair, high cheekbones, and almond-shaped eyes. Her skin was dark and her figure petite. She caught the attention of every man who crossed her path, but she had eyes only for my father. Soon after they met, he married her and brought her from her native Mexico to the United States. They settled in San Francisco, where my sister, Lesley, and I were born.

The late sixties were a trying time for all Americans, but even more so for my mother, who knew hardly any English. Her relationship with my father was challenging, and, eventually, the language barrier drove a wedge between them. What finally separated them for good was my father's alcoholism. He was an angry and oftentimes a violent drunk.

By the time my brother, David, was born in 1974, my mother had grown tired of the endless fighting and my father's drunken binges. She now had three small kids, very little money, and a husband who hardly ever stayed home. When he did, my mother only felt worse.

We had glimpses of the man I knew my father could have been, if not for the demon that possessed him—which is how I chose to look at it. Unfortunately, those glimpses were few and far between, so my sister and I often hoped that he wouldn't come home at all.

As I grew up, I fought to control whatever I could in my life, but the chaos often seemed unbearable. At ten years old, I found solace in the same addiction that consumed my father: alcohol. I now knew *why* my father had drunk so much. Alcohol allowed me to escape. It let me be comfortable in my skin, something I never was.

At age thirteen, I became obsessed with my weight. For every pound I lost, I felt as if I had deposited one more dollar in the bank (I was banking against my own insecurity). The skinnier I became, the better I felt about myself. Weight was the only thing I could control. By simply focusing on my weight and the caloric content of every known food, I could escape everything else that was a mess in my life.

I had so many reasons to self-destruct: my father's unpredictable and explosive behavior, kids hurling racial insults at me and, worse, calling me fat. I started to blame and resent my mother for being Mexican. By the time I was in high school, I had already embarked on a path to self-destruction.

I drank every day, all day, and, not surprisingly, was flunking my classes. Then, as if to torture myself further, I began to binge and purge. I ate whatever food I desired and then purged it by taking laxatives, throwing up, or even overexercising.

In 1985, within a month of graduating high school (which I'm sure happened only because the teachers never wanted to see me again), I left home. A few times I even found myself homeless, but I was unwilling to go home. My life was on a downward spiral.

In 1988, a friend told me about a place that could help me, a place with people just like me—Alcoholics Anonymous. When I walked into my first meeting, I felt like I had come home. The members didn't judge me; they accepted me, with no questions asked. For the first time in my life, I felt comfortable in my own skin.

My life seemed to be turning around. I enrolled in college, began working, and stayed sober, but one thing still haunted me: food. I needed it to live, and it was the only vice I had left. I couldn't simply put it on the shelf and not deal with it. Food was a temptation I had to confront every day of my life.

Still, I managed to keep my eating disorder under control. I was determined to keep moving forward and "trudging the road of happy destiny," as they say in AA. This happiness, however, would be short-lived. By 1995, the juxtapositions within my life were jarring.

The effects of the eating disorder monster had really started to show, yet I was newly married to Kristoff St. John, the accomplished Emmy award–winning star of the soap opera *The Young and the Restless* and the father of our two gorgeous children, Julian and Paris. Our lives seemed perfect.

We'd met when I was twenty-one and he was twenty-two. At the time, he was acting in the sitcom *Charlie and Company* with Gladys Knight and Flip Wilson. When I first met Kristoff, I tried to play it cool. I pretended not to know who he was, but, of course, I did know him, because my sister watched his show every week and was in love with him. I called her immediately after meeting Kristoff and said, "I just met the man I'm going to marry and have kids with."

By that time, I knew that when I put my mind to something, I could make it happen. We were impulsive kids who fell in love and planned our first child after only two weeks of knowing each other. Being crazy in love, we didn't worry that the odds of our marriage surviving were almost nil.

By 1996, Kristoff filed for divorce. He would be the second-most important man in my life to leave me.

I had just graduated from college with a BA in psychology, and although my relationship with Kristoff was tempestuous, the thought of divorce left me feeling powerless. I started to have severe panic attacks, and my compulsions got even more obsessive. I began to starve myself. It didn't matter that I was only twenty-nine years old and weighed about 115 pounds, that many people considered me beautiful enough to pay me to model, that I had a black belt in Tae Kwon Do, and that for the last eight years, I had been sober. None of that mattered. When I woke up every morning, I felt old, fat, ugly, and powerless.

In an attempt to control my weight, I tried to subsist on a diet consisting almost entirely of chicken breasts. Not surprisingly, these attempts at self-control resulted in a complete loss of control. I always began each purging cycle with the foods I craved—burgers, French fries, ice cream, and doughnuts—followed by lots of water to help me purge. The cycle was never ending: binge-purge, binge-purge, until the spiraling brought me to the lowest point in my life.

I found myself locked in the bathroom, trying to escape voices in my head brought on by extreme anxiety. In utter despair, I thought that death seemed better than living in this nightmare.

Then I heard a knock on the door. I didn't know whether it was imaginary or real. Fortunately, it was real. It was Kristoff, the man I thought had abandoned me. He convinced me to go with him, and he got me admitted into a hospital for people with eating disorders and psychiatric troubles.

I spent the next four weeks there, as the doctors tried to figure out whether I was suffering from obsessive compulsive disorder (OCD), bulimia/anorexia, panic disorder, or generalized anxiety disorder (GED). Take your pick—it was all of those and more.

When I left the hospital, I realized that my addictions and disorders were not the result of how I *looked* but rather of how I *felt*. I knew I needed to really find myself. Who was I? What was true happiness for me? My gift to myself was to make a plan.

I wanted to live the life I wanted, to be the best me that I could be. It sounds easy to say, but how many of us live the lives we want? How many times have you wondered, How did I get here? To make a plan, we must first ask ourselves, What do we want for ourselves?

At that time, however, I continued to juggle acting classes, auditions, and amateur Tae Kwon Do tournaments. Much to the annoyance of my acting coach, I often showed up late to class because of Tae Kwon Do training.

Finally, my exasperated acting coach asked, "Do you want to be a fighter or an actor?"

Without taking even a moment to rationalize, I let my heart speak for me. "I want to be a fighter," I said and walked out.

That decision put me on *my* path. In that moment, I unconsciously decided that I'd rather be happy and poor, as long as I could do what I loved. I've never looked back since.

What I dreamed, what I saw in my mind, I decided I would become.

My dad, in one of his few moments of sobriety, told me that if I pretended to be someone long enough, I would eventually become that person. I wanted to be known around the world as a fighter, and who better to help me become this than Don King? People told me I was insane for thinking that Don King would sign an unknown and, worse yet, a fighter from the martial arts who had no boxing experience! But I had been through hell and back; at this point, rejection was nothing to me.

I sent King my photo and résumé. In 1997, he signed me. So, I kept on envisioning my life as I wanted it to be. I dreamed of opening for Oscar de la Hoya and being on pay-per-view, fighting in front of thousands of fans. In 1998, I left King for his rival, Bob Arum. I spent the next three years opening for Oscar de la Hoya on the biggest boxing cards of the decade.

I dreamed of becoming a world champion. And on June 12, 2005, I became the IFBA Lightweight Champion of the World. In November 1999, Hugh Hefner made me the first boxer ever to grace the cover of *Playboy* magazine, which proved that being Mexicana was beautiful after all, and being curvy was not so bad either. On June 14, 2008, two weeks shy of my forty-first birthday, I became the WBC Welterweight International Champion.

Today, I am twenty years sober, still fighting, and in the best shape of my life. More important, I *love* me exactly how I am.

I hope my story can inspire you, to conquer your dreams and know that *nothing* is impossible. My mother always reminded me of what Cesar Chavez used to say: "Si se puede!" (It can be done.) Envision yourself as the beautiful, fit, healthy, smart, successful woman you have always wanted to be, and one day, you *will* be that person. Then you'll realize that you always *were* her.

ACKNOWLEDGMENTS

I want to thank my son, Julian, and my daughter, Paris, for brightening up my world. And thanks to all of the people who made this book possible: my mother, Socorro; my agent, Frank Weimann; writer Robert Wolff; WBC president Jose Sulaiman, WBC executive secretary Mauricio Sulaiman, and WBC's Jill Diamond for giving me the opportunity to become a WBC champion; Tim Elliott and Eric Manlunas, the producers of *Million Dollar Workout*; everyone at Wiley; everyone at the Literary Group International; and finally, my ex-husband, Kristoff St. John, my sister, Lesley, and my brother, David, for inspiring this idea.

Getting into Fighting Shape

Imagine waking up most mornings feeling good about yourself and your body. When you look in the mirror, you like what you see. Instead of zeroing in on the fine lines, gray hairs, or rolls of fat that perhaps no one but you notices, you actually see yourself for who you really are—a powerful, invincible woman.

Imagine walking into your kitchen carrying this sense of power with you like a shield. Imagine seeing all sorts of fattening, delicious foods around you—doughnuts, cake, and bagels and cream cheese. You might hear these foods whisper to you, but they do not call to you as loudly or convincingly as usual. You overcome any urges to eat these foods and instead choose to eat a scrambled egg-white breakfast, one that will fuel your body and your mind.

You're still as busy as usual. You still have your job and kids and hobbies. The basic facts of your life have not changed. Yet, on this imaginary morning, you do not allow your stress, busyness, and responsibilities to penetrate the shield that protects your best interests.

You somehow, for once, manage to put your needs at the top of the to-do list. You fit in that workout that you seem to keep putting off. You shower, then slip into those pants in the back of your closet that used to feel too tight. You feel fantastic. You feel calm. You feel in control of your life.

With *The Knockout Workout*, this imaginary morning can become an everyday experience. You can wake each day feeling beautiful, sexy, and powerful. The plan goes a step further than most weight-loss plans.

Like many fitness and weight-loss systems, this program helps you to lose weight and build a better, healthier, and sexier body. The boxing-inspired fitness routine will without a doubt transform your body—lifting your butt, shaping your shoulders, flattening your tummy, and revving up your metabolism.

Yet, unlike any other weight-loss system, the Knockout Workout also teaches you how to feel healthier and sexier in your body. The workout teaches you how to create this inner sense of power, the one that allows you to, without fail, complete those workouts, eat those foods, and generally stay on course to create and live in your best body and your best life. You will love it.

If you ask my mother, she will tell you, "Mia was born a fighter." That's probably true. I remember two altercations from my childhood: one at the grammar school playground, the other at a high school football game, both the reaction to relentless racial slurs directed at my Mexican American heritage. I'll just say that the girls who started the fights ended up looking a little different afterward.

I had a lot of struggles in my life, and fighting was something that no one could take away from me. Not only has fighting been something I've done all my life, but it's been one of the great loves in my life.

I started Tae Kwon Do at age six. I quit for a few years and did not become a black belt until my twenties. After graduating from college, I competed in tournaments for many years before making the switch to boxing. While I loved Tae Kwon Do, boxing gave me a way to express my passion for fighting and make a living from it at the same time.

I started my boxing career in 1996 and turned pro at twenty-nine. I really learned to fight on national television. My mother was concerned at first about me being in boxing, but she knew it was something I loved, and she has always been my biggest fan.

In 1997, during my first professional fight, I knocked out my opponent in just fifty-four seconds. I didn't have much experience when I began boxing, but I got a lot of attention, even at the start.

Everybody criticized me. I was too feminine. I didn't fit the image most people wanted of a woman boxer. But I didn't want to look like a man.

There are two sides to me. Even though I do have masculine interests, I do have a lot of feminine interests as well. I want to be a boxer and stay feminine despite some people's old belief that women should stay in the kitchen and cook.

My earliest boxing mentor and my first trainer was a man named Art Lovett. Art trained me in a Los Angeles park, because at the time most boxing gyms in the city wouldn't allow a female fighter to train in their gyms. Art passed away during my third pro fight in 1997, but he continued to coach me through every fight even after he was gone; his spirit has always remained alive with me.

One of my reasons for leaving the legendary Don King for boxing promoter Bob Arum was that Arum understood how important it was for me to be seen as a strong Mexican American woman. Arum knew who I was as a Latina, and he understood the importance of boxing as a Mexican sport and what I wanted and needed for my image to inspire others.

This was one of the reasons I chose to do *Playboy*. I couldn't pass up the chance to bring attention to women's boxing, inspire other Latinas, and let people know that you can be a professional boxer as well as a vibrant and sexy woman—and more important, not look like a stick figure! I was the first boxer and one of the few Mexican Americans on the cover of *Playboy*, and to me and many other people that was a major victory.

In the course of my boxing career, I've been fortunate to have fought on the undercards of some of the most popular names in boxing: Oscar de la Hoya, Roy Jones, Antonio Tarver, and Arturo Gatti. They were some of the biggest fights ever, and it makes me smile to think that years from now, I will be able to say I was a part of them.

People always ask me what it feels like to be a professional fighter. For one, it's been an amazing experience. On fight night, it's so overwhelming, because when you take that walk from the dressing room through the tunnel to the ring, with twenty thousand fans screaming and cameras and lights in your face, you have to think of yourself as an entertainer. My mind-set is that this is a job and I'm here to perform. Otherwise, it would become too overwhelming. You feel like you're going to the gallows. If you get knocked out, you're getting knocked out on national television, and there's nothing worse.

When it comes to feeling pain in the ring, I don't feel a thing. My adrenaline is going so fast. However, the next morning I feel everything, and it's painful.

Coming off of that adrenaline high after a fight is horrible. It's a nightmare. It usually takes a few days to get over it, and then you're okay. If you win, it's even harder to recover because you're so high emotionally when you win that you come crashing down when it's all over.

I think the most difficult thing to deal with is that boxing is a painful sport emotionally. Your goal is to hurt somebody so badly that you knock them unconscious. Of course, when I win and knock somebody out, I jump all over the ring. But then I leave feeling a little bit of heartache.

One of the hardest parts of boxing is leaving the dressing room, walking through the tunnel, and entering the ring. It's petrifying. No matter if you win or not, you're still going to get hit. But after I get into the ring, the bell rings, and the first punch is thrown, all fear is gone.

I'm very close to my mother, my brother, and my sister. My mother is always in my corner when I fight. I wouldn't want to fight without her there. When I'm in the ring and I see my opponent, I think, "I'm gonna have to knock this person out," because I don't want my mother to worry about me.

My mom's such a big fan that she'll get mad if she sees me during a fight with my jab down. She'll yell, "Keep your left hand up!" She's always right there as my coach. And I'm telling you, nothing slips by her, be it my fighting, my diet, my routine—anything!

I still go into the ring with the mentality that I'm going to win no matter what. But do I go in there willing to die? No. That's totally changed. I'm not like that anymore.

I go in there now as a boxer with a lot more strategy that has come from experience and maturity. When I was young, I went into the ring wanting to destroy the opponent no matter how I had to do it. Now when I go in there, I'm very strategic.

Many times, people ask me what lessons I have learned as a boxer. Besides avoiding getting knocked out, there are many. Fighting has taught me about humility, compassion, respect, acceptance, perseverance, and that in this thing called life, whatever happens to you, you just keep moving forward with your goals and dreams—no matter what.

As much as I love boxing, it isn't my whole life. I have to juggle my career and my kids all the time. Since having two wonderful children, I know what it is like to have to lose that after-pregnancy baby fat. With two kids to take care of, I also know what it feels like to have no time to work out.

Being a woman, I know what a big deal image and weight issues can be. For a boxer, our weight is public record, so imagine what it would be like having to always get on a scale on weigh-in day in nothing but a bikini and having your weight announced to a crowd of photographers and TV cameras.

So relax. You won't have to go through such pressures with this book. In fact, it's going to take the pressure *off* of you and put *power* in its place by giving you the knockout strategies that are going to make you look and feel fantastic!

Once we feel in control of our lives, we no longer obsess on the one thing we feel we can't control—our weight. I've come to realize that I only feel fat when my life feels out of control and when things in life happen that I am powerless over. That realization helped me to see myself and my life differently, and it gave me back control of my life, my career, and my happiness. And as I rebuilt myself into a happier, stronger, and more powerful version of my former self, I found myself taking many risks and making unconventional choices.

When I made the decision to become a professional boxer, I quickly discovered that the training I put into boxing transformed my body and my mind. Through boxing, I confronted many roadblocks—roadblocks that had prevented me from living up to my potential as a mother, a daughter, and a person.

Each time I hit the bag, walked into the ring, and wielded punches against an opponent, I confronted my fears and strengthened my confidence. I confronted the roadblocks that kept me from feeling good about myself and confident about my abilities, the roadblocks that prevented me from living life—*really* living life.

Now, more than ten years later, I have emerged a different woman—one with unwavering inner power. I look beautiful on the outside and feel beautiful on the inside. I have a healthy relationship with food, with exercise, and with my body.

I want you to know this feeling. I want you to know that it is possible to shed the shackles that lead to low self-esteem, poor body image, and self-sabotaging eating habits. I want you to discover the sexy, confident, powerful version of yourself. I want you to have access to the tools that can not only reshape your body and transform your health, but also put you in control of the biggest determining factor of your health and well-being—yourself.

The Knockout Workout takes the empowering life lessons that I have learned during more than ten years as a boxer and puts them into a simple, easy-to-implement plan, one that will help you build a lean, fit, and powerful body by first and foremost creating a powerful mind. *The Knockout Workout* will help you transform your health, body, and life no matter the reasons for overeating and underexercising.

You need not have been diagnosed with an eating disorder to know what it feels like to lose control. To understand the importance of this concept, think about your own life and your own issues with food and exercise. You may not ever have binged, purged, or excessively restricted your calories, but you probably—at one time or another—have faced the sense of powerlessness that can erode willpower, determination, and motivation.

Powerlessness leads to giving up. Powerlessness makes you skip your workout. Powerlessness makes you eat the fries and burger when you really wanted to eat the grilled chicken salad. Powerlessness makes you wallow in self-pity. Powerlessness leads to you looking in the mirror and seeing a fatter, uglier version of yourself staring back.

I'm willing to bet that you know what to eat and how to exercise. The plethora of health magazines, Internet sites, and news shows do not keep healthful living a secret. You may already know about the importance of eating more lean protein and vegetables and less saturated fat and processed carbs. You may already know about cardio, about weight training, and about stretching. Your problem is making it happen on a consistent basis.

In *The Knockout Workout*, I'm going to give you the tools to consistently eat healthfully and exercise daily, without fail. In this groundbreaking plan, you will strengthen your motivation by learning how to train and think as professional female boxers do. This total lifestyle change will help you to fight the motivational roadblocks that prevent you from putting yourself first, from loving your body, and from consistently striving to achieve your best potential.

The Knockout Workout helps you build inner power by teaching you how to train your inner fighter. The lessons you will learn will help you to defeat myriad opponents—some human, some not—that block you from living your most healthful, happy life. These opponents differ from person to person and include:

- Bad relationships
- The stress of motherhood
- A busy career and home life
- A dysfunctional work environment

You may have heard of—or even tried—other boxing-inspired programs. Perhaps you've taken kickboxing classes or followed boxing-inspired fitness videos. If this is the case, then you have already experienced a taste of the type of workout you will complete in *The Knockout Workout*. Yet this plan is more than a series of kicks and punches that will shape your legs, butt, and shoulders as you rev up your heart rate and burn fat. Indeed, it's much more than that.

On this plan, you will build an inner sense of power and use that power to improve every aspect of your life. Specifically, you will learn how to:

- Use exercise as a form of therapy
- Deal with the real roadblocks in life rather than using them as excuses to self-destruct
- Eat for strength

Research shows that people who exercise regularly do so not only to burn calories and tone their bodies; they do it because exercise makes them *feel* good. In *The Knockout Workout* you will learn to love exercise not only because you will complete interesting, invigorating, body-changing workouts, but also because you will learn how to use exercise to satisfy your inner need for fantasy, challenge, curiosity, and control. For example, by envisioning yourself boxing imaginary opponents (in the form of real people, health problems, or life challenges), you will be able to continually motivate yourself.

Many studies have linked poor body image—how you view yourself when you look in the mirror—with poor eating habits, lack of exercise, and weight gain. Many people think that weight loss automatically improves body image, but I can tell you from experience that successful weight loss requires the reverse. You must improve your body image by improving your sense of power over the world around you. Only then will you be able to lose weight and keep it off.

With the Knockout Workout you will learn to pinpoint the real reasons you feel fat, old, and ugly. (Hint: they have nothing to do with what you look like in the mirror.) You will also learn mental strategies—strategies that I've used inside and outside the ring—to deal with the situations that threaten your sense of inner power.

You will follow a meal plan that maximizes lean protein (fish and chicken), whole grains (oatmeal and brown rice), green vegetables (broccoli and spinach), and other wholesome foods. Although you will learn how to avoid your personal trigger foods—the ones that erode your sense of inner power when you eat them—you will still be able to eat delicious foods. For example, I still eat dark chocolate and natural ice cream. Every healthful nutrition plan should include your favorite foods, and *The Knockout Workout* will teach you how to include yours without ever losing control again.

All told, this 1-2-3 combination works effectively to create a knockout body and mind. You will be doing some great workouts that I personally designed, to shape your arms, lift your buns, firm your thighs, and shrink your waistline.

You'll eat foods that help to build the muscle that will speed your metabolism and create a sexy shape to your body. Most important, you'll find the tools you need to wake up every morning and look in the mirror and see a beautiful, sexy, youthful you—no matter your age.

Step

1

THE
FOUNDATION

1

Looking and Feeling Great

Before you picked up this book, you may have tried diet after diet and dozens of exercise plans, yet nothing seemed to click. Believe me, I know the feeling.

Even though I'm a professional boxer, I can't begin to tell you how many years it took me to find just the right combination of workouts, nutrition, and mental discipline that would bring me the greatest happiness and give the best results. You can discover these secrets the easy way. I'll save you years of trial and error, frustration and disappointment, and will give you only the tools that work, and work well.

First, I want you to change your attitude about transforming your body. You can start by thinking of exercise as something that's fun, something you really look forward to (and believe me, you will, once you start seeing and feeling all of the positive changes in your body). Throw out your old concept of exercise; visualize it as something healthy that you do each day, just like brushing your teeth.

Get comfortable with the idea that exercise will be a fun-filled part of your day. It's how you'll live each day for the rest of your life. No hurries, no worries, no deadlines—just moving your body in a way that makes you feel good. You'll be amazed at the results.

Turning Struggles into Success

We all struggle through tough times, don't we? For so many of us, life just never seems to get easier. Relationships, family, friends, career, our bodies, food, exercise—it can all be such a challenge. Yet if you change your outlook, each obstacle can become a stepping-stone to a new you and a better life in the future.

Truly, it's amazing how we each find our own path. I used the anger and frustration in my life and directed them toward fighting through Tae Kwon Do. Not only did I become a black belt and a competitive fighter, but I gained an incredible amount of discipline and self-respect at the same time.

Perhaps your path involves using this book, which has come into your life at a perfect time to help you change your thinking, your diet, and your exercising and completely turn your life around. I want you to know that I've been there, and I understand what it's like to struggle. So, smile. Relax and be kind to yourself from this moment on, while I help and guide you.

Let's Take a Trip Together

You're about to embark on an exciting journey. Let's call it our little road trip, one that will finally put you in control of your body, your eating habits, your fitness regimen, and your life.

On this trip, you will learn how to knock out the obstacles that have been standing in your way, the temptations that call your name from the freezer or the fridge, and the urge to procrastinate that convinces you to skip your workout in exchange for a nap.

Many people think of these as demons in their lives that they constantly struggle against. But to me, calling them demons gives them too much power, because once you see and understand them for what they are, they lose *all* of their power.

Let's be honest: many of us fight against thoughts and influences that can (and often do) hold us back every day. My personal struggle came in the form of an eating disorder, one that caused me to binge and then purge. It was a tough thing to go through, but like all of the other struggles in my life, I looked it square in the eyes and determined that I would understand why I let this compulsion control me and where it came from. I would seek help for it and then live the rest of my life free of it.

Your struggles (which affect your body and your life) may come in a milder form. Yet so many times, the root cause is the same. Often, it's simply a trigger that causes you to lose control over your fork or spoon and your physical exercise. It feels like powerlessness and creates a very familiar cycle:

1. Something happens—an event or a series of events—in your life that causes you to doubt yourself, lowers your self-esteem, or makes you look at yourself in a way that brings you unhappiness, and this chain reaction starts to erode your sense of inner power.

2. As the negative thought cycle continues (after all, you keep thinking about it, right?), the negative events, images, and feelings in your life manifest in ways that make you feel bad.

3. Because you keep everything bottled up inside, these negative influences and bad feelings gain more power.

4. You begin to see yourself in ways that make you unhappy. Instead of realizing what a beautiful person you are, you replace that self-image with one of ugliness.

5. As your self-esteem and self-worth plummet (after all, you keep dwelling on all of the things you don't want or that don't bring you happiness, right?), you feel a loss of control in your life.

6. To make yourself feel better (if only for a short time), you eat more, sleep more, watch more TV, party more, exercise less (or

exercise more, to an unhealthy extreme), or indulge in other self-destructive behaviors that make your guilt feelings stronger, increase your unhappiness and feelings of being ugly, and drain the inner power you so desperately want back but that is nowhere to be found. The cycle just keeps going and going and going.

But that was then, and this is today! I'm about to give you that power back, and much more. You will learn not only how to change your body, your eating habits, and your appearance, but also how to think like a fighter, a knockout champion, with the mental toughness and the physical strength that will keep you feeling great, looking great, and in control of your life.

Together, we'll embark on an exciting trip that will change your body and your life. I'll share with you the essential elements of the training plan I used to get into peak boxing shape.

The Three-Pronged Approach for Changing How You Look and Feel

Without a doubt, I know this plan will help you reach the physical and mental destination you've always dreamed of, and on the way there, you will tap into an inner power and strength you never knew you had. It will help you achieve your happiest and highest potential. Just how will you do this? You'll learn a three-pronged approach that encompasses diet, fitness, and your mind.

Diet

When I use the word *diet*, I simply mean a lifelong eating plan and not a temporary fix. In the past, you've probably tried the "Drop 7 Pounds in 7 Days" diet, or variations thereof. And you learned the hard way that there is no such thing as a quick fix. It's time to forget the hype and grab hold of methods that work.

The reason people so often fail at dieting is that they approach it the wrong way. They either look at it as a quick fix (that is, "I've got to drop two dress sizes in two weeks"), and when they get off the diet, they go back to their old way of eating. Or else they take the diet to an extreme and do way too much for too long. I see this often, especially here in Los Angeles, where people think image is *everything.* It usually goes like this: A woman who has struggled with her weight and body image for many years finally hits on a diet approach that brings better results than all of the other plans she's tried in the past. So, she sets a target goal of wanting to get down to a specific weight or drop *x* number of pounds. She tells herself that once she hits that target, she'll be happy.

Lo and behold, after a few months or many, she finally achieves her goal, but instead of stopping there and enjoying her success and her new body, she can't. She's now getting attention and compliments from other people for the first time in her life—or maybe it has just been so long since she last heard compliments, she can't remember. All of this gives her a quick shot of self-esteem and fuels her motivation to continue dieting. She convinces herself that she still needs to drop a few more pounds to really feel good about herself.

So, she makes her diet even stricter and denies herself the foods her body is craving. She hears her family's and friends' compliments turn into worry and concerns, yet despite these warnings she begins to lose control. Fear, the fear of stopping and backsliding to the way she used to look, has now set in.

She sees herself with different eyes than when she began her adventure many months ago. Now, she sees herself as lacking. She feels a constant need to change her body so that it will live up to the perfect image she has in mind today. Yet this image, this goal, will change tomorrow and will keep changing the next week and the week after that. This type of thinking, belief system, and behavior will take her to one destination: Eating Disorder Avenue.

Some women are able to see what is happening and catch themselves before they arrive. Others refuse to see and hear the messages they receive, both internally and externally, and they soon discover that Eating Disorder Avenue can be a long one-way street, *unless* they can turn themselves around and head in the opposite direction.

But these are the very issues you will *not* have to worry about or even think about as you read this book and follow my plan. You will always have the power to be in control of your body, your eating, and your life. You have my word on it.

The Knockout Workout plan includes foods (and many of my favorite recipes and meals) that will fuel your workouts, promote your body's lean muscle, help boost your metabolism, and keep your body fat at the ideal level. Yet my plan also allows you to eat delicious foods. Even though I watch my diet during the week, I *love* to occasionally indulge in Mexican food, chocolate, and ice cream. With my plan, you'll be able to enjoy your favorite foods, too.

At the end of the day, if whatever you're doing isn't fun or enjoyable (as exercising and eating well should be), you won't get excited about it or do it for very long. My plan is big on fun and big on results!

Fitness

The word *fitness*, depending on your past experiences, will either bring a smile to your face or make you feel uneasy. What does *fitness* mean to you?

The Greeks believed that life was movement and the more you moved, the greater the life you would experience and enjoy. In the Knockout Workout plan, the movements you'll do won't involve heavy weights, complicated exercises, or unpleasant visits to a sweaty gym. You'll learn some great moves that are specifically targeted to your body and the results you want to achieve.

Like dieting, fitness can either be a curse or a blessing, depending on how you do it. For me, it's always been a joy, even when I was training intensely for boxing championships. Exercise and working out have always made me feel good.

Whether it be climbing stairs, taking walks, moving around the house and the yard, or going to a gym for a workout, as long as I'm moving my body in some way, regardless of how little or how much time I spend doing it, I'm a happy woman.

Again, it all goes back to what I said earlier: you need to make exercise a no-brainer part of your everyday life (like brushing your teeth). When you do, then as long as you're moving (those Greeks knew what they were talking about), you will be doing good things for your mind, your body, and your health.

Women need to know how important strength training is for overall health. Training with weights keeps your muscles strong and your bones healthy. The more muscle you create, the more fat you'll burn. It's the best antiaging medicine I know! There is nothing wrong with trying to look fit while you work out. When you look in the mirrors at the gym, you will feel better about yourself. This will inspire you to work hard, especially as time goes on and you start to see results.

I work out five or six days a week. Sometimes I do less, sometimes more; for example, I may decide only to run if I feel really tired or maybe I'll just walk or lift weights or box. The point is, I keep moving. Every day I move. It relaxes my mind and helps me feel better about myself. I'm not trying to achieve a perfect body, because that will never happen. I have stretch marks and cellulite, as many women do.

Over the years, people have asked how I train my body. When I train for a fight, I focus less on weights and more on traditional boxing exercises. In between fights, I train more like a bodybuilder, using heavier weights with less repetitions to build muscle and strength. I also keep my cardio training to a minimum.

Although it's true that cardio workouts such as running on a treadmill will help you lose weight, people are often surprised when I tell them that I don't think you need to spend hours on a treadmill every day to look good. I think it's more beneficial to increase your pace for 20 to 30 minutes and burn more calories in a shorter amount of time. And doing fast-paced cardio exercise four times a week will give you great health benefits and keep you in fantastic shape.

Over the years, you have undoubtedly read, seen, or heard many conflicting "facts" about exercise and diet. A lot of them were probably accurate, but others may have been confusing or untrue. Before we go any further, let me and my good friend Robert Wolff destroy some of the myths and the misconceptions you might still believe about exercise and diet, so that when we get into the fun stuff that's coming up, you'll have a clean slate.

Mind

Your mind-set is what puts everything together in your life. It's your center of belief, your engine of action. If you believe something is possible for you to achieve, then you will find a way to make whatever you desire a reality.

For any obstacle that you face in life, use your imagination and pretend that you are a champion boxer. Think of any tough situation as if you are in the ring, pushing against your opponent, and neither of you will budge. This merely wears you out, and no one gets anywhere. Yet if you simply "let go" and step to the side, whatever opposes you will fall forward, giving you the upper hand.

Fighting is mental and requires a lot of strategy; life itself is not so different. You fight better when you are relaxed and have a clear mind. It's the same process for attaining your goals and dreams. You visualize what you want before you step into the ring, you see the end result you want to achieve, and you keep thinking about that success over and over, each and every day, until it happens.

A boxer can have the greatest natural gifts, strengths, conditioning, and abilities, yet if he or she doesn't have it mentally, that boxer will get beaten every time. This is why the best boxers are always thinking and strategizing. They replay their best moments and pre-play their future moments for how they want things to happen. That's what I want you to do.

Start to see yourself as a world-champion fighter and think like one. Feel the confidence and joy that this mind-set brings you. See and feel yourself in a new body, with a new look and sensation: a perfect version of yourself.

Let the image soak into your mind, as you see your body perfectly sculpted with just the right amount of muscle and strength. Imagine what you look and feel like when you have all of the endurance, conditioning, and energy you could ever want, whenever you need it. This peak mental and physical state allows you to perform every activity you did in the past, only better. In addition, you have now arrived at a place in your life where you can perform any other activity, with ease, that you could only dream of doing in the past.

In other words, I want you to see, visualize, imagine, and feel yourself and your body as already having arrived in the place you want it to be. Don't think about it as a future event that will require months and months of hard work to achieve. Imagine that all of the hard work has already been done, and right now you are enjoying these incredible feelings.

I'll soon tell you about my favorite mental conditioners. I know you'll really like them and that they will work wonders for you. But for now, just keep this in mind: scientists have proved that your mind doesn't know the difference between a real and an imagined event. Studies performed on elite athletes have shown that the same muscle fibers that are used by athletes who physically do a sport are also prompted into action by the athlete merely thinking about doing his or her sport.

This means that when I tell you to see your body's peak fitness as something that already exists right now, you're sending your brain the same signal that you would if your body had already arrived at the goal. By pre-playing your success mentally as something that has already occurred, you give your brain the commands it needs to make all of the necessary changes in your beliefs, ideas, and actions that will take you to your goal in the fastest, most direct way possible. And it'll almost feel effortless.

You Can Do It, and You *Can* Get There from Here

Yes, you'll be eating better. Sure, you'll be exercising more effectively, and doing all of this requires that you take action. But the joy and excitement you'll feel as you take charge of your diet and your exercise won't feel like work in the least.

You'll see and feel results, day by day, little by little, inch by inch, until you reach your goal. Just remember that when I began Tae Kwon Do, boxing, and working out, I started at the same place you did—as a beginner.

2

Dispelling the Myths

Let's talk about some of the fitness myths that have been around for so long. Where these myths came from is anybody's guess, but one thing's for sure, people still recite and accept them as fact, and it's high time we changed that. Here are twenty-four of the most absurd ones.

Myth #1: I need to exercise a lot.

Who started this? You don't need to exercise a lot unless you feel the need to always be doing something. The actual amount of exercise time that's necessary to give you great results is very little. It's not a matter of how long you work out, it's what you do when you work out.

If you do endless set after set and exercise after exercise but aren't doing the *right kind* of exercise for your body and without the *right intensity*, then much of your time and effort is wasted.

Once you start doing the exercises that are best for you, and you learn to make your body work more effectively simply by changing how you do these exercises, you'll see major improvements. In other words, you'll get better results in less time. Stay tuned for a few pages, and I'll show you how.

Myth #2: I'm too old to change the way I look and feel.

Says who? Scientists and researchers? Not a chance. Their studies show that everyone, young and old, can greatly benefit from exercising. Even people in their nineties can get stronger and build muscle.

This myth was started by individuals who were either too lazy to get off their butts or too frustrated after blindly following the wrong advice and information for so many years.

The truth is, if you have even the slightest desire to look and feel better, you will be able to do this. Your desire to change some things in your life already puts you halfway to the finish line. Follow the instructions in this book, and you'll cross it quickly and with ease.

Myth #3: I need to have expensive equipment or to join a gym to change how I look and feel.

Do you own a pair of tennis or athletic shoes? Good. Put them on, head out the door, and start walking. You'll be doing the same thing and gaining the same health benefits as people who walk on expensive treadmills, climb stair machines, or pedal fancy bikes.

If you've got two arms and two legs, then you've got all the equipment you need to exercise your body. I've even met people without the full use of their arms and legs who have great-looking, healthy bodies because they used what they had and used it well.

You'll soon discover that it doesn't take high-tech equipment to achieve high-quality results.

Myth #4: With so much information, I'm confused about what I should do.

I know what you mean. I'm going to help you find the information you need to transform your body, your goals, and your life. It'll be fun and easy.

Before you begin, imagine pouring clean water through your mind to wash away all of the dirt and the sludge that have accumulated over the years caused by beliefs that have held you back. As I talk about changing how you look and feel, stay open to everything that you find interesting and might like to try. Don't get attached to believing that one way of training is better than another, because once you do, you close your mind to all of the other possibilities that might work for you. Let me explain.

Some people believe that you must work out three or more times a week to get the best results, but what if you can work out only two times a week, yet you're still getting great results? Just because you're not able to work out on that third day, does that mean your program is less than successful? Of course not.

Others believe that you must lift heavy weights to exercise productively and effectively, or else you're simply wasting your time. So does this mean that if you use lighter weights or no weights at all, then you've simply wasted your time on nonproductive exercise? Not if it makes you feel good, physically and emotionally.

Still other people say that full-range or short-range movements are the best, and they can cite myriad reasons. So, does that mean if you used one type of movement instead of the other, you didn't exercise correctly? Of course not.

Use both kinds of movement. Better yet, try anything and everything that keeps you excited, interested, motivated, and happy. Use all of the methods, but don't get locked into any one type of exercise. Keep an open mind about everything.

Myth #5: I need to eat all the time and buy expensive supplements if I'm ever going to change my body.

Chances are, if you've read this in magazines, especially the muscle, bodybuilding, and fitness publications, there's a good reason: those magazines stay in business because they sell supplements. Some magazines have their own private brands, and they also let competing supplement companies advertise in their publications to create ad revenue. Other magazines don't sell their own supplements but have pages filled with ads from companies that do. So it's in their best interests to promote supplements, and it's not necessarily in yours to buy them.

If you're eating nutritious foods, drinking plenty of water, getting enough sleep, and exercising regularly, then the only supplement you might wish to take would be a good multivitamin/mineral capsule and perhaps a few others that I'll tell you about in the nutrition section of this book. Unless you have a psychological need to eat all the time, then don't do it. A world-champion athlete once said, "I know people say to eat five or six small meals a day, but I just can't do it. I always eat a good breakfast, lunch, and dinner, and if I can add a healthy snack at night, then I do it. If not, no big deal."

We're all different, and when it comes to your own nutritional requirements, simply give your body what it needs and not what someone else says you should have. Later in the book I'll provide some helpful guidelines for you to follow.

Myth #6: I've tried so many diets and exercise plans over the years; I'm so frustrated that now I don't believe anything will work.

That's great news! Through trial and error, you've discovered what won't work, and you're closer than ever to learning what will. Everything in life can teach you a valuable lesson if you simply keep your mind open and look for the lesson contained in each experience. Think of it like this: Your goal is to look and feel better. So, you have a final destination—an end point—you wish to reach. You buy books, magazines, videos, equipment, and the like, all in hopes that they will help you reach your destination.

Somewhere along the way, however, something doesn't work, and because you're trying so many different things at once, you're not really able to tell what works and what doesn't. So, you come to the quick conclusion that none of it works and you give up, frustrated, yet again.

Let's change all of that. After you finish this book, you'll know what works for you, and oftentimes only a slight adjustment in how you do things may finally produce the great results you've wanted. After all, many times the difference between a million-dollar race horse and one that doesn't win major races or big money is only a split second in timing.

For you, this means it doesn't take much to win big in changing how you look and feel. Often, you'll need to make only small adjustments to give your body exactly what it requires to change quickly. Stay on the racetrack, my thoroughbred friend, and I'll take you to the winner's circle.

Myth #7: One machine is all I need to have great abs or a great body.

The people who keep selling those ab machines on TV are misleading you. It's so easy to be lured into thinking that if only you buy their machine, you'll look like those models. But did you ever notice the fine-print disclaimer at the bottom of the TV screen that appears when the announcer tells you how to order? It usually says something like this: "Results shown here are not typical" and "Blah . . . blah . . . blah . . . along with diet and exercise." Meaning, the male and female models who demonstrate how to use the machines didn't get their midsections and their bodies to look great only by using those machines.

You can bet your last dollar that they spent many months, even years, working out at gyms and following strict diets, not to mention that they were blessed in the genetics department. But somehow, the actors don't mention this while you are watching them crunch or slide forward and backward.

The truth is, you don't need any machine to help you look and feel great, so save your money.

Myth #8: I'm afraid if I get started and miss any workouts, I'll lose what I've worked so hard for.

It's human nature, isn't it? The fear of losing something. Take a good look at your life, and see how much this fear influences what you do and don't do. If you're like most people, you'll be shocked.

Let's begin by thinking about what you'll gain from exercising and eating right, how much fun it will be, and how great it will make you look and feel. And let's put this whole exercise-eating thing in perspective.

Exercise was something you did naturally as a kid; now you must resolve to do it for the rest of your life. Consider it a daily activity, like eating, sleeping, or brushing your hair. Don't you remember when you were a kid how good you felt when you played hard all day and came in at night and slept like a bear in hibernation? Your body was growing and was lean, you could eat and eat and still not get full, you were healthy, and, most of all, you were happy.

Just because you're a few years older—okay, maybe many years older, big deal—doesn't mean this has to change. Sure, the kind of exercise you do and the time you have to do it may be different, but the great feelings produced by exercising and being active can always be a part of your life.

The health benefits that result from physical activity and a healthful diet accumulate over many months and years, and they stay with you. Whenever you miss a workout or spend days or weeks not eating the most nutritious foods, don't worry about it. Simply do your best to start your regimen again as soon as possible, and you'll be fine.

Our society lives by instant results and also believes in instant failure. Both beliefs will only propel you along a dead-end road that leads to misery, frustration, and unhappiness. It's time for you to get off this road.

Here's some advice that will put your on again/off again discipline in proper perspective. Remember that all of those days, weeks, and months of no exercise and lousy eating will stop the very instant you begin exercising again and eating something nutritious. That exact moment is the end of the old way; the new way has begun. Each day, build on your progress, little by little, and you'll quickly reach your goal.

Myth #9: Working out will make me too tight, too stiff, too big, or too slow.

People who don't work out are the ones who typically say this, because if they did work out, they'd know what a load of hooey these statements are.

Working out will help you perform every physical action better than you could if you didn't exercise. Your body is designed to be worked. Years ago, most of our ancestors made their living from physically working hard.

In modern times, that's not the rule; it's the exception. So, does this mean our bodies have changed and, along with this, their need to be exercised? Not a chance. We need physical exercise even more now, because so few of us actually do much beyond get up, stand in the shower or sit in the tub, get into the car, sit at our desks at work, and walk from the car to the movie theater, the food store, or the mall and then come home.

You don't need to become a world-class athlete—unless, of course, you want to—but simply someone who gives her body a little regular exercise. Don't worry; what you're about to learn won't make you too big, too small, too thin, too slow, too tight, or too anything else. It *will* make you too terrific, but I have a feeling you'll be able to handle that.

Myth #10: Only certain people can have great-looking, healthy bodies.

Why do people continue to believe this nonsense? And why do we deny ourselves so many wonderful things, such as having great-looking, healthy bodies? It's almost as if we get a perverse pleasure from neglecting whatever is good for us and avoiding what we want most.

If you're reading this, that means you're alive, and if you're alive, this is the only prerequisite to your looking and feeling great. So relax, you've already passed the test. The rest is easy.

Most people fall into the trap of thinking that unless they can look like the most popular model, actor, or athlete, it's pointless to make any effort to improve themselves. So they get depressed and frustrated and lose the desire to look and feel their best.

It's as if this model or actress has become the new gold standard—and the standard always changes—by which they judge themselves and their appearance. Naturally, no matter what they do or how hard they try, they will always fall short of their ideal.

You are the only one who has your body and your look. No one else does. And if you are smart, you'll be proud of this and play it to the hilt, just as these celebrities do. That means no one could ever look like you. Now, if you're following where I'm going with this, it should make you smile, because in this world we all want to feel special and unique. And if you exercise and eat right and follow the tips I'm about to share with you, you will have a great-looking, healthy body for the rest of your life. Compare? Don't you dare. Simply focus on being your own personal best.

Myth #11: I really can't do much to change my body.

Who told you that? One thing I can guarantee is that if you don't do anything, you most definitely won't change your body, unless you call getting more out of shape a change.

Each of us has her own uniquely shaped body, and even though we're human, we're all a little different. Genetics plays a big role in how you'll ultimately look. I've met people who were so genetically blessed that their bodies gave the impression that they were elite athletes, yet they did little, if any, training. I've also met others who have busted their butts for years, working out and eating right, and the best they can do is keep the pounds off and maintain a halfway decent shape.

So, are you doomed if you have less-than-desirable genes? Heck, no. By doing the right exercises for your body and eating the most nutritious foods, you can sculpt your body to its optimal shape and can attain the look and the physical well-being of someone who is extraordinarily healthy and fit.

You can do a lot to change how you look and feel today, and reading this book is a good place to start.

Myth #12: I need to eat a lot of protein.

Be careful of "experts" who say that only their way of eating is the best. You'd be surprised to learn that many of these experts (doctors, scientists, researchers, and the like) are actually a bit flabby or out of shape and have less-than-desirable, unhealthy-looking physiques themselves.

Protein is an essential nutrient that your body needs each day. Yet so are carbohydrates and fats. Remember that we're talking about balance here—not too much of one or too little of another nutrient, but a balance of all three types.

A lot of people don't get enough protein (the good kind, such as fish, lean beef, chicken, turkey, eggs, and nonfat dairy products like skim milk, yogurt, and cottage cheese). Then they wonder why their bodies look and feel the way they do. Their diets are haphazard at best.

The human body thrives on regularity. It wants to be fed, watered, exercised, and rested regularly, and your body performs wonderfully when you take care of it this way. The problem arises when you don't, and instead try to find miracle cures that you hope will make up for your neglect.

Myth #13: I need to eat a lot of carbs.

Read myth number 12. I will say that many people eat far too many carbs compared to the amount of protein in their diets. Whether a carb comes from fruit, vegetables, or grains, your digestion ultimately breaks it down into a sugar. The body has a tendency to store too much sugar as excess body fat, especially if you're not burning those sugars at work, by being active, or while exercising.

By all means, give your body a good balance of carbohydrates from fresh vegetables, some grains, and fruits, but don't overdo it. And pay close attention to how your body reacts to carbohydrates.

If, after you've begun this exercise and eating plan, you find that you're having a hard time losing that last bit of body fat, cut your total number of calories back a bit, and make those reductions primarily in carbohydrates. See if that doesn't help.

Myth #14: Finding the best workout for my body will be too difficult.

Human beings are is basically lazy. Admit it, don't we want to find the magic exercise, pill, or diet that will be "the one" that will change us?

The vast majority of people don't take enough time to find exercises that work best for *their* bodies. Instead, they page through magazines, listen to friends, and watch the latest fitness guru on TV, and presto chango, they're right back where they started.

You're the only one who has your body, your level of experience, your goals and dreams, your genetics, and your desire and level of commitment, and only you can know what works best for your body. Sure, other people can suggest things, but free advice is worth about as much as it costs you, which is nothing. By all means, though, try their advice to see whether you can find exercises that you like and that will work, and then do them.

Myth #15: I'm afraid I'll fail.

The fear of failure has kept more people from living the lives they've always dreamed about but were too afraid to try. And it's the same for working out and changing how you look and feel.

Every human who has walked this earth has suffered failures, shortcomings, adversities, and disappointments. These experiences are meant to teach us valuable lessons, and life will keep repeating these lessons—albeit in different ways—until we finally learn them.

Consider failure something to look forward to, because failure is feedback. It's probably telling you that your plan may be good, but it needs to be changed a bit in order to work and bring success. You don't scold a baby or think it is stupid just because the child falls down when it's learning how to stand and walk. We were all babies who failed while learning to walk, but it wasn't too long before we mastered this activity, and we've been doing it perfectly ever since.

If your exercise or nutrition plan isn't working the way you want it to, begin by changing only a *few* things at a time until you find the right combination that works for you. Anyone who's ever built a great body or achieved a goal has also failed many times before succeeding. The world is filled with women and men whose lives prove that the bigger the failure, the bigger the ultimate success. You can't have one without experiencing the other.

Myth #16: I'm afraid the beneficial results won't continue.

I can tell you that at first, good results will come very quickly, because if it's been a while since you've gotten yourself in shape, then your body is receptive and responsive to any training. You'll find, however, as does everyone who works out, that the results do slow down. That's normal, so don't sweat it. Look at it this way: when the results start to slow down, it means your body is getting stronger, tighter, and more in shape.

The body responds very quickly to the demands placed on it. If you give it good workouts, eat right, and get plenty of rest, it will respond beautifully. And if you want it to keep responding that way, you must vary the activities you ask it to perform. Your body habituates—that is, it gets used to the same old thing—very fast, and one of the best ways to catch it off-guard is to give it something new and different to do each time you work out.

Think about it: if you do the same old barbell curls with the same weight during each workout, do you really think your arms will ever get stronger? Hardly. Your arms grew stronger months ago when you first started doing those curls with that particular weight, and unless you change your arm workouts, the weights used, and so on, then you're only spinning your wheels by hoping your arms will continue to respond to this workout.

Keep your workouts fresh and novel, and your body will reward you with great results, month after month and year after year.

Myth #17: Working out is too complicated. How can I ever know if what I'm doing is right?

All of the "experts" have helped perpetuate this myth. I mean, c'mon, look at all of the books, magazines, TV shows, and infomercials that proclaim their way, their machine, and their supplement to be the best. With so much information, who and what can you believe?

The simple way is still the best way. Build your foundation and your workouts with the basic barbell, dumbbell, and bodyweight-only exercises. These are the rocks on which your body will stand, and the waves and the wind of other exercise fads will not crumble it or blow it away.

Good results are the only evidence you'll need to judge whether you're doing effective workouts. Some people measure results by how much weight they can lift at once or over a given period of time. For others, their appearance determines whether the program is a success. And for many others, it's simply a matter of how they feel. If working out makes them feel better and reduces stress, they enjoy it, and it adds quality to their lives, then their exercise program is an out-of-the-park home-run success.

Pick a method to determine whether you're getting results that make you feel good. When your fitness program needs a few changes, make them immediately. Begin by changing only one or two things at a time until you're again enjoying the results that are most important to you.

Myth #18: I need to work out at least three times a week to get results.

This is not true. Does the body actually benefit most from training every other day, such as three days a week? I've yet to see a conclusive, exhaustive study that covers all of the bases and every extenuating circumstance: the number of days one can train, all of the workouts one can do and their various intensity levels, every type of person who trains and his or her experience level, and the amount of time needed for maximal recuperation (physiological, neuromuscular, and mental). Without a study like this, no one can state definitively that three days per week of training is the absolute best method anyone can use.

Most training methods have their benefits and drawbacks. The key to ultimate well-rounded training success is to incorporate some aspects of each method to make your workout ideal for your body, your goals, and your experience and lifestyle.

If three days a week works for you, then do it. If it doesn't, keep changing it until you find the type of training that really rings your bell. Even if it's only walking, the most important thing is that you do some type of physical activity every day. It's a positive habit that'll keep you looking and feeling great for life.

Myth #19: Because their bodies are different, men and women must work out differently.

Who started this myth? Besides the obvious size and strength differences, are they saying that men and women have different arms and legs? Don't both genders have two of each and don't those muscles get stronger, tighter, firmer, and bigger from weight training?

Sure, for esthetic reasons, women tend to stay away from heavy squats and dead lifts, simply because these two exercises tend to thicken the body structure. This, however, doesn't mean that a woman wouldn't get great results from the exercises.

Many of the dictates of how a man or a woman should train come from our inner need to conform our lives and bodies to the whims of what society deems acceptable, sexy, attractive, masculine, feminine, and so on, and have little do with how a woman's or a man's body would respond to the same exercises.

Train the way you want to, and forget about what society or anyone thinks or says you should do. Ultimately, you're the only one who walks around inside your skin and who knows what makes you happy.

Myth #20: Losing weight will make me healthier.

On the surface, this myth appears to be true. But notice the word *weight.* It should say, "Losing *fat* will make me healthier." You see, most people equate fitness and success in dieting with simply losing weight. But this isn't necessarily true.

If a person loses too much weight, there's a good chance she is also losing valuable lean muscle tissue. Much of the fat we have is basically inert. It doesn't do much; it just sits there and takes up space. Does that mean all fat is bad? Heavens no, for your body needs a certain amount of fat to keep it healthy, protect your organs, and so on. The problem is *excessive* fat.

Lean tissue, on the other hand, is living tissue that needs nutrients to sustain it. This means food, and the more lean tissue one has—within reason, of course—the more calories the body will burn. Think of it like this: lean tissue helps to keep your metabolism running, and fat slows it down.

If you want to lose weight, try to lose fat instead of simply weight. Set a goal to lose one-half to one pound of fat per week. This is very doable, and it's a healthy goal for most women and men. Remember that a pound of fat has 3,500 calories, and to lose one pound a week, you'll need to either burn 500 extra calories a day or cut out 500 calories a day. One of the fastest and easiest ways to lose a pound a week is to do a combination of both; reduce your food consumption by 250 calories a day and increase your activity so that you burn an extra 250 calories a day.

The number on the scale means nothing. Besides, muscle weighs more than fat, and it looks so much better! What's most important is whether you like what you see in the mirror. Let this be your guide, and you'll do just fine.

Myth #21: I don't want to lift weights because I'm afraid I'll get too bulky.

This is one of the biggest myths I hear from women, and it's not true! Believe me, it would take years of hard lifting and dieting, not to mention plenty of supplements, to really bulk up. It just won't happen, unless you get lucky. Putting on muscle was the hardest thing I have ever had to do. Putting on fat, no problem, but adding muscle is *hard* work.

Most women do not realize this. They think that spending hours on the treadmill is the way to go. If you don't mind staying flabby, that's fine, but if you like the well-toned look, then weights are a must. Plus, it's important to keep your muscles and bones strong as you age.

Myth #22: I want to lose the fat first; then I'll lift weights.

You need to realize something very important: building muscle will help you burn fat much faster! And with better muscle tone, you're going to look better. So throw your scale away. It's not how much you weigh, it's what you look like that counts. Remember that muscle weighs more than fat, so stop thinking about your weight number and aim to lose inches.

Myth #23: I just can't find the time to exercise.

I understand that working all day in an office can be mentally draining. So relax, you don't have to join a gym.

Go for a run or a walk around your neighborhood for cardio; do push-ups (with your hands far apart for the chest and close together for the triceps); dips on a park bench or a chair; calf raises on a step; walking lunges, squats, and abs anywhere; pull-ups on the monkey bars; jump rope anywhere; shadowbox anywhere; and kick anywhere. There is so much you can do if you just improvise a little.

I always keep a pair of dumbbells at my house just in case I am too tired to go to a gym. Many times, I'm out of town and the hotel doesn't have a gym. So I might do bodyweight-only exercises in my room, go for a walk or a run, or climb the stairs for a few minutes at a brisk pace.

The point is, just move, no matter what. You'll sleep better, feel better, and look better. How you feel on the inside always shows on the outside.

Myth #24: Latinos rarely work out.

Who started this myth? It is so untrue! My Spanish-speaking friends tell me it's hard because most of the gyms have classes in English only and most tapes and CDs are in English as well.

I spent many years doing Tae Kwon Do before I turned pro in boxing, and that is where I learned the most important lessons in my life. My coach always told me to give everything 100 percent or don't do it at all (not that I've always lived up to that, but I do try at all times). He told me to always respect my opponents (in and out of the ring). He taught me not to feel sorry for myself and to take back control whenever I feel victimized. And I learned those lessons (and more) because I worked out.

The Knockout Workouts

Okay, enough of the myths. Let's get down to the business of helping you look and feel fantastic! Let me tell you what kind of workouts you'll be doing in the Knockout Workout plan.

I firmly believe that boxing is one of the best and most effective workouts you can do. You're burning calories and toning your muscles at the same time. Each round in this workout consists of three exercises, with a speed round in between to really get your heart rate going. You'll also stretch and rest between rounds to loosen up any sore muscles.

You'll perform some great boxing-style motions such as punches and kicks. Even though you won't use weights (only your arms and legs), you'll be amazed at what a fabulous workout these boxing movements are.

I'll have you do some speed rounds to keep your heart rate up during certain exercises and workouts. You'll be surprised to discover how picking up the tempo will give your body greater conditioning and power, whether it's from speeding up your punches, kicks, twists, and walking, or decreasing the rest time between sets, reps, and body parts. We'll do some exercises with weights and some without. Most important, we'll keep the workouts fresh, exciting, and fun, to produce the best results.

For some exercises, you will need some light hand weights. You will also need a padded floor or an exercise mat. Some execises require gym equipment, but there is always an alternative exercise that doesn't require any special equipment.

I learned early on in my boxing and Tae Kwon Do training that if you copy the successful ways of another person (of course, adapting them to your own body and goals), then you, too, will become successful that much quicker. That's how I want you to use these tools. The exercises, workouts, and routines I'll give you contain only the moves that work, and work very well.

Feel free to adapt and change things for your body, in whatever way works and feels best for you. I encourage this. But I want you to do the core movements just as I describe and show you, so that you'll get the quickest and best results possible. In thirty days, you and your body will be happy that you did.

3

Your Personal Challenges

We all have challenges in our lives. They're simply a part of living and learning. I think you'll agree, however, that recognizing or admitting these challenges can make us a little uncomfortable. The good news is that there are many techniques we can use to mentally overcome any challenge or roadblock that gets in our way.

Personally, I found that the boxing ring was my way to put the challenges I faced into a concrete form. Let me explain. Whenever I walked into the ring for each fight, I faced a given opponent. But actually there was more than one. There was the physical opponent I saw standing across from me on the other side of the canvas, and there was the mental opponent—my challenge—that I visualized morphing into my physical opponent.

My challenges in life enabled me to fight, but I was never angry at my opponent. A good fighter looks at the bout like a game, always anticipating her opponent's next move. If she guesses right, there is no better feeling in the world. If she guesses wrong, it really is like the old saying "the agony of defeat"—it is true agony!

Getting mad at your opponent means you've lost control, which results in your not being able to think clearly. As a result, you'll most likely lose the fight. I fought this way early in my career when I was very green. When I became a better fighter, I never let my emotions take over. You'll soon learn to do the same.

Okay, now it's time to get honest. You may have a long list of challenges that have kept you looking and feeling the way you do, or you might have only one or two. Either way, the fact remains that you do have challenges, and that's what you're going to knock out.

If you're like most of us, you might be aware of some of them but not all of them. So, let's speed things up and bring them to the surface of your awareness, where you can see them, understand them, and conquer them.

Take some time to reflect on the following questions:

- When you feel fat, ugly, or old (or all three), what circumstances are affecting your life?
- What in your life makes you feel powerless?
- What gets in your way of making healthy changes for the better?

Write down on a sheet of paper whatever comes to your mind. Don't edit it. Write it all down. Do you have the answers? Good! Let's move on.

Now think about all of the times you struggled through these challenges; try to remember events or outside circumstances that triggered your feelings of losing inner power. Think about the kinds of foods and lifestyle choices that may have either made your problems worse or temporarily given you comfort from them.

Here's what I discovered about myself. Whenever I ate foods made from white flour—pasta, doughnuts, pizza—I felt sluggish and powerless. When I thought about this, it dawned on me that I've always had a tough time controlling my intake of these foods. I loved them! Yet it took me many years to learn the reason for this.

Nutrition experts and psychologists call these foods "trigger foods," and they may be playing a huge role in how good you look and feel, inside and out. The good news is that with my eating plan, you can still eat delicious foods, but you will want to keep a lid on the trigger foods that make you feel powerless.

Along with food choices as a challenge you might face, there are others that almost sneak in the back door and take hold of your life before you even realize the damage they're doing and the power you've given them over your health and appearance.

Overconsumption of Alcohol

Like anything in excess, too much alcohol won't help your body look and feel its best. Personally, I don't drink, but I know that many people do enjoy a drink or two. That's not a problem. Numerous studies have shown that drinking a glass or two of red wine daily can have health benefits (just as dark chocolate does).

The problem begins when you find yourself "needing" a drink to get through the day, to deal with stress and frustration. So much so, that you feel powerless without it. Now, that's when alcohol *is* the problem.

Yet I want you to consider something else: the fact that too much alcohol can really slow and impede the benefits your body receives from exercise and a good diet. Robert Wolff describes this in his book *Bodybuilding 201*:

Researchers from the University of California have shown that less than 5% of the alcohol calories you drink are turned into fat. Rather, the main effect of alcohol is to reduce the amount of fat your body burns for energy.

Successful weight loss is all about oxidizing (or burning) more calories than you eat. When they go on a diet, many people choose low-calorie alcoholic drinks, mainly because they contain fewer alcohol calories than their regular counterparts. However, this recent study, published in the *American Journal of Clinical Nutrition,* shows that even a very small amount of alcohol has a large impact on fat metabolism.

In the study, eight men were given two drinks of vodka and lemonade separated by 30 minutes. Each drink contained just under 90 calories. Fat metabolism was measured before and after consumption of the drink. For several hours after drinking the vodka, whole body lipid oxidation (a measure of how much fat your body is burning) dropped by a massive 73 percent.

Here's why.

Rather than getting stored as fat, the main fate of alcohol is conversion into a substance called acetate. In fact, blood levels of acetate after drinking the vodka were 2.5 times higher than normal. And it appears this sharp rise in acetate puts the brakes on fat loss.

A car engine typically uses only one source of fuel. Your body, on the other hand, draws from a number of different energy sources, such as carbohydrate, fat, and protein. To a certain extent, the source of fuel your body uses is dictated by its availability.

In other words, your body tends to use whatever you feed it. Consequently, when acetate levels rise, your body simply burns more acetate, and less fat.

In essence, acetate pushes fat to the back of the queue. So, to summarize and review, here's what happens to fat metabolism after the odd drink or two.

1. A small portion of the alcohol is converted into fat.
2. Your liver then converts most of the alcohol into acetate.
3. The acetate is then released into your bloodstream, and replaces fat as a source of fuel.

Your body's response to alcohol is very similar to the way it deals with excess carbohydrate. Although carbohydrate can be converted directly into fat, one of the main effects of overfeeding with carbohydrate is that it simply replaces fat as a source of energy.

That's why any type of diet, whether it's high-fat, high-protein, or high-carbohydrate, can lead to a gain in weight. So the bottom line is that even a small amount of alcohol (this study used two servings of vodka and lemonade) can have a big impact on the rate at which your body burns fat—even if the drink is low in calories.

Just keep all of this in mind as we look at the challenges that have been holding you back in the past and what you'd like to change from this day forward.

The Savior Syndrome (Always Saying "Yes" to Requests for Your Time)

My goodness, name one woman who hasn't experienced this at some point in her life! We love to help others. It benefits them and makes us feel good inside, knowing we made a difference and hopefully made someone's life a little better. This is all well and good. But the problem isn't that we help others; it's what happens when we can't say no.

You have only 24 hours (1,440 minutes) each and every day. You've got a life. You've got goals, dreams, desires, and ambitions. You want to experience life and learn from and enjoy it, right? Of course you do.

I know what it's like to be a caretaker. All moms know this, but we also have to take time out for ourselves, even if it means getting someone to watch the kids so we can meditate, work out, do yoga, or simply have lunch with a friend. As moms, we have a really hard time saying no to our kids, but we have to do it. We need to make time for ourselves; otherwise, we become stressed and take it out on our kids. Who wants a cranky mom, right?

The problem comes when you find yourself giving up too much of your time to the requests and needs of others. If you try to cut back on these obligations, it triggers your feelings of guilt. But this is exactly when saying yes is the wrong thing to do. You need to create boundaries so that you are not overwhelmed by taking care of others. Again, whenever you feel swamped with caretaking duties, just take a step back from your life. Get out that sheet of paper and write down all of the reasons you feel compelled, pulled, or forced to say yes to others, even when deep down you don't want to. You'll discover your triggers, and once you see them clearly, right in front of you, then the power that you've given away (by saying yes, yes, yes, so often) comes back into your life.

What always gives me great strength is realizing that I wasn't upset by things that actually happened in my life as much as I was by my perception of what I thought was happening. In other words, the event by itself contained no emotion. It was simply an event that happened.

It was my perceptions, however, and the labels I attached to events in my life that made me feel either happy or sad, good or bad. Recognizing this about the people, the conversations, and the events in my life immediately infused me with power and control and destroyed the triggers that had given me problems. Before I learned to think differently about challenges, I had always worked so hard to get rid of them, yet in frustration could never overcome them. Looking at my life from a different perspective changed everything for me, and I know it can do the same for you.

Control Issues

Why do we care so much about what others think of us? Why do we think we need to exert control over the actions, words, and behaviors of other people? Have you ever given this much thought? Are you a control freak, one who needs to know in advance how this or that will turn out before you even take the first step? If you answered yes, then you and I need to talk.

Just this element alone, the need for control, can be one of the biggest triggers and challenges in your life, if you don't stop for a moment to understand how it has limited you in every way.

My favorite thing to repeat to myself is the Serenity Prayer: "God grant me the serenity to accept the things I cannot change, the courage to change the things I can, and the wisdom to know the difference." I say this prayer often. I also use meditation to help me relax and visualize my plan. I remind myself every day of all the things I am grateful for. I tell myself that I love myself every day, despite all of my flaws. I give back as much as I can to people who are less fortunate than I am. These powerful little sayings and thoughts help release my inner pressures and make me feel so much better.

I want you to admit this, right here and right now: the only person you will *ever* be able to control is you. Period. End of story. Other people will live their lives, follow their own paths, and do their own thing, regardless of what you say or do and whether you like it or not.

For goodness' sake, let them! They were given their lives to live as they desire and you were given yours to do with it as you want. That's the beauty of this thing called life: each of us is given this blessed gift to create and experience anything we desire—no limits!

Once you step back (are you still keeping that sheet of paper nearby?) and look at all of the hours, days, months, and years you've wasted feeling frustrated and disappointed at what others said or did, you'll realize just how silly you were to fixate on these things. Let's change all of that.

You can overcome your need to control everything by realizing that when you demand others to act a certain way or do or say a certain thing just so you can feel good inside, you're asking them to lie to you. You're asking them not to be who and what they are, but instead to become who you think they should be—all to meet some need you believe you have or to make you feel good for a brief moment.

That, my friend, is keeping it as "unreal" as it gets. Whether it's a lover, family, friends, a business colleague, or whoever, just let these people go and let them *be*! When we spend too much time focusing on others, it's really because we don't want to focus on ourselves. It's a diversion from our own problems.

And about all of the other things in your life that you think you must control—guess again! Even the most successful people agree that although you may plan, take action, and never give up in pursuing your goals, at the end of the day people and events operate on their own schedules. You cannot control everything, no matter how hard you try. You need to accept that whatever happens will happen when the time is right.

So, relax. Start enjoying your life again. It's supposed to be fun!

THE KNOCKOUT PLAN

4

Knockout Workouts

The Knockout Workout will help you sculpt a powerful, lean, and sexy body in the shortest amount of time. By incorporating speed rounds into your workouts, you will boost your heart rate and burn fat while you build curvaceous, metabolism-boosting muscle.

These speed rounds mimic my training program for boxing. During each workout, you will push yourself in 2- to 3-minute sprints/rounds, taking short 30-second to 1-minute breaks to recover. Each workout includes a warm-up, stretches, and a cooldown.

Hitting the Bag

This efficient cardio and toning workout shapes your entire body, especially your shoulders and legs. You will need a heavy bag (freestanding

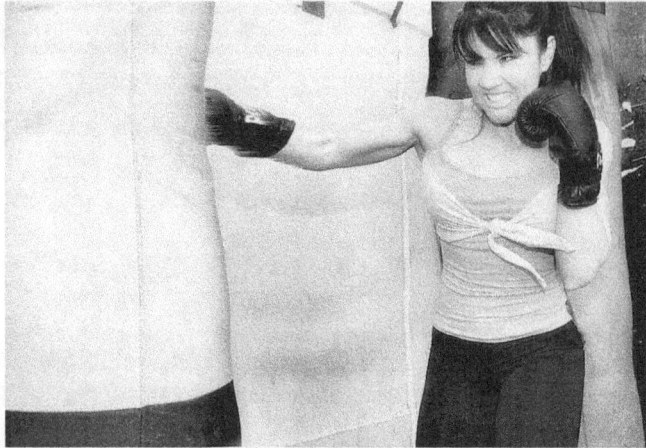

or hanging) and a speed bag. During this heart-pumping routine of kicks and hits, you will push yourself to your personal limit, creating a sense of accomplishment and confidence.

As you attack the bag, visualize yourself battling your personal challenges, which will build the inner strength and power you need to face those challenges in real life. During your 30-second to 1-minute rest periods between rounds, you'll catch your breath by bouncing on the balls of your feet.

I like to use the heavy bag to practice punches and the speed bag for hand-eye coordination. When you hit the bag for cardio, make sure you wrap your hands with a pair of boxing hand wraps and wear a good pair of gloves weighing no less than 8 ounces.

Start with 4 rounds, 3 minutes each, with 1 minute of rest, then increase to 6, 8, and 10 rounds. If you're in awesome shape, you can have 30 seconds of rest.

If you want to make this your only workout of the day, throw in some leg work and kick the bag 10 times per round with each leg, then go back to punching. Stay on your toes at all times to challenge yourself. You will find this is a grueling workout. Make sure you have some great upbeat music to listen to (I always wear headphones when I do this exercise), and wear an outfit you like. It will help build your confidence and make you feel attractive.

The Jab/Right Punch

THE MOVE

This move consists of the two most basic punches in boxing: a jab/right punch. Many in boxing believe that the jab is one of the most important punches in a boxer's arsenal, if not *the* most important one. Boxing legends such as Muhammad Ali were famous for defeating opponents by using the jab punch.

The jab/right punch is an easy boxing move to execute if you remember a few key things.

HOW TO DO IT

Get your body in the "ready fight" position by keeping your body upright with the feet facing forward. Bend your knees slightly. Put your chin down, keep your elbows bent, and keep your arms up with both fists close to the sides of your face.

As you extend your left arm forward for the jab, you will twist it like a corkscrew. The palm of your hand faces your cheek when you begin the move, and as the arm extends forward and away from the body, the hand will twist until the arm is fully extended and the palm faces the floor at full extension. Also, as you extend your right arm forward to execute the straight punch, the right side of your upper body will twist and turn toward the punch, thereby giving you more power.

The breathing cadence will be *exhale* as you *execute* the punch and *inhale* as you *return* the arm and body back to the starting position.

Footwork and arm and upper body coordination are very important for the jab/right punch.

The lead jab punch (that is, the right or left arm, whichever you punch with first) is always followed by that same side's lead foot. A right jab punch is followed by the right lead foot coming forward.

So let's put it all together and see how it will work. A right hander (for a left hander, simply reverse the moves) will start with the left hand executing the jab and will punch directly ahead, keeping the elbows in close to the body.

As you jab punch forward, your left foot will follow by taking a step forward. Your right foot will turn slightly clockwise. After executing the jab, the body should now be facing slightly open and to the right.

As you recoil and bring back the left arm (the one that jabbed), extend your right hand out to punch and at the same time, turn your upper body *into* the punch. As you do so, your right back foot will now be facing forward as you lean slightly forward with your knees bent.

After you've thrown the straight right punch, recoil and bring back the straight right punching arm and return to the starting jab position. Repeat this 15 to 20 times in rapid motion and without locking your elbows during any of the punches.

Hooks and Uppercuts

THE MOVE

Hooks and uppercuts are two of the most difficult punches in boxing to execute effectively, but don't get discouraged because we are here to get into shape. For that purpose, these punches are much easier. Imagine that your hooks are being thrown to either side of someone's head; the most commonly thrown punch is the left hook, to counter the opponent's jab. Hooks to the sides of the body are used as well. Now imagine your uppercuts are being thrown directly under someone's chin. It can be a dangerous punch to throw in the ring, but outside of the ring it feels awesome because it really works your inner delts. I love using this punch, especially with weights, before a fight.

HOW TO DO IT

Hooks: Stand facing forward in your boxing stance, feet shoulder width apart, with your left foot in front and your right foot in back. If you are left-handed, simply reverse this stance. Turning to the right, bring your left hook across your body to the right. So your left hand and bent elbow comes up and over and across. Your lead foot pivots in the direction of the punch. You back foot remains pointing clockwise. Recoil the punch back to starting position. Rotate your hips to the left, bringing your right hand and bent elbow up, over, and across to the left. Your back leg now pivots slightly to the right in the same direction of the punch.

Uppercuts: Remain in your boxing stance. With your fists by your cheeks, rotate your hips to the left, bending just slightly down. The left fist now comes up as if to land underneath your opponent's chin; the body follows in the direction of the punch. The feet remain in position. Recoil back to the starting position. Rotate to the right, slightly bending downward, and come up with the right uppercut, underneath the chin of your opponent. Recoil back to the starting position.

PUTTING IT ALL TOGETHER

Alternate left hook then right hook, left uppercut then right uppercut. Really twist your body, especially when you're doing those uppercuts. Be sure to squeeze your abs during this one. In boxing, you're always working your abs, no matter what you're doing. Let's do this for 60 seconds now that you have it down.

Boxing-Inspired Weight Lifting

For the body-sculpting workout detailed in this chapter and in chapter 8, you will use light hand weights, lifting and lowering them at a fast cadence. (For more on how to figure out the right size of weights for you, see the list in the section called "My Favorite Weight-Training Exercises" in chapter 8.) Completing 25 to 30 repetitions per exercise, you'll move quickly through a series of my unique signature moves: squats with bob and weave, dumbbell uppercuts, standing dumbbell jab-rights, lying dumbbell jab-rights, and sit-ups with a punch and a jab.

This weight-lifting routine mirrors my in-season training regimen; it starts with a shadow-boxing warm-up, followed by stretching. Then you'll move into my series of boxing-inspired signature moves, interspersed with traditional weight-lifting moves such as dead lifts, dumbbell rows, walking lunges, hamstring curls, crunches, and leg lifts.

All told, you will sculpt your body from head to toe, paying special attention to moves that will lift and shape your butt and firm and flatten your tummy.

Cardio Rounds

During these sessions, you will engage in your favorite form of cardio (running, power walking, stair climbing, jumping rope), splitting your session into 2- to 3-minute speed rounds interspersed with 30-second to 1-minute breaks at a slower pace.

Level One Workout with the Knockout

As a mother of two, I know you don't have all day to train, so I designed this workout for anyone. All you need is 30 minutes. It's simple and fun. Knock it out, and you will get great results.

Each workout at Level One lasts 4 rounds (the shortest number of rounds in a women's boxing match) of roughly 15 minutes in total duration.

Are you ready? Let's go and burn some calories!

The Warm-Up

For the warm-up round, I recommend that you use a jump rope, but if you don't have one at home, that's okay, just jump without it. You're still going to burn calories, and you'll still break a sweat. This round is about 60 seconds long, and you're just going to get your blood flowing. This warm-up is one of the best workouts in boxing and is one of my favorites, too. You'll concentrate on burning calories and toning muscles, and, most of all, you'll have fun.

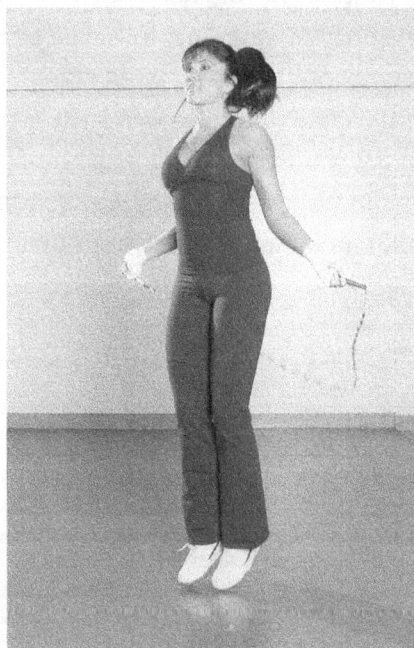

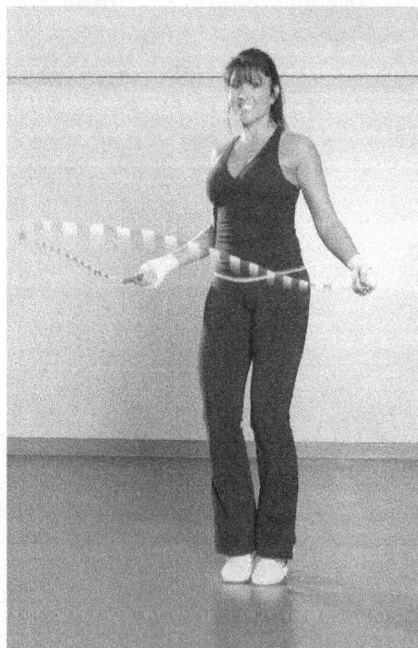

If you are jumping without a rope, hold your hands near your hips as you would if you were holding the rope. Pretend you are actually turning the rope so that your wrists move. Remember to keep breathing while you're jumping. Sometimes you forget about your breathing, and that's one of the most important things a boxer can be aware of.

After you've finished your jumping warm-up, you'll go into the hip rotations.

Hip Rotations

THE MOVE

I use hip rotations as part of my warm-up and stretching, simply to loosen up my body. This is especially important in boxing, because we rotate our hips with every punch. I like to rotate my hips as far as I possibly can without injuring myself. By keeping your stomach tight, you will be able to feel it even in your abs.

HOW TO DO IT

Stand facing forward, with your feet shoulder-width apart. Bring your hands up in the boxing stance, fists by your cheeks as if to protect your face, with your elbows bent. Rotate your upper body and hips to the left as far as you can, keeping your legs facing forward, then switch and rotate to the right as far as you can. You're going to do this for about 30 seconds. Make sure you really squeeze your abs while you're twisting. Pay attention to your breathing; you may find that it feels best to inhale when you are facing forward and to exhale when you have rotated to either your left or your right, because that sideways movement compresses your diaphragm, squeezing the air out.

Punch Time

THE MOVE

Before boxers execute their punches, they put their bodies in the proper punching position that allows them maximum effectiveness. That means paying close attention to where the hands, the arms, the torso, the lower body, and the feet are placed. Anyone can throw a punch, but it's the best boxers who know it takes coordinated timing and body position working together to make that punch effective. Here's how I want you to get your body ready for punching.

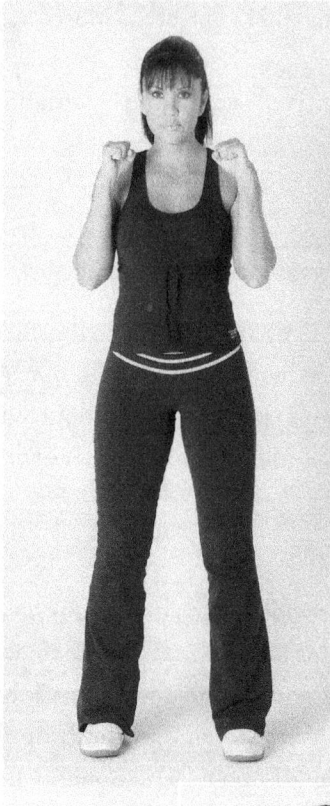

HOW TO DO IT

Stand with your shoulders relaxed and your abs pulled in, and bend your knees slightly. With your elbows bent, make a fist with each hand and hold your hands in front of your face, around cheek level. Your feet should be shoulder width apart.

You'll turn your body slightly sideways in both directions when you punch so that you'll get a greater stretch. First turn your body to the left and punch with your right hand. As you extend your right arm into a punch, keep your abs tight. Pull that arm back to the starting position. Then switch by turning your body to the right and punching with your left arm and then pull it back quickly. Your feet will remain in the same position, so the move becomes a slight twist. Make sure your shoulders stay relaxed—they should not be up by your ears. Really extend your punches out there, and keep that elbow and arm straight. Alternate jabs for a total of 25 to 50.

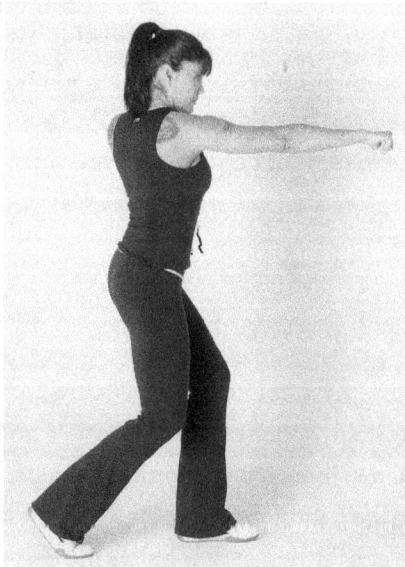

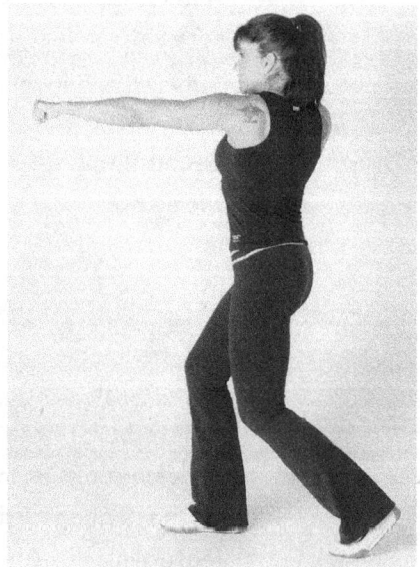

Arm Stretches

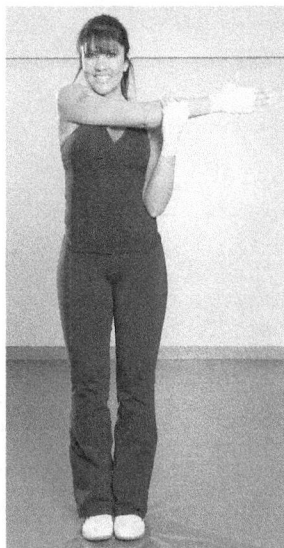

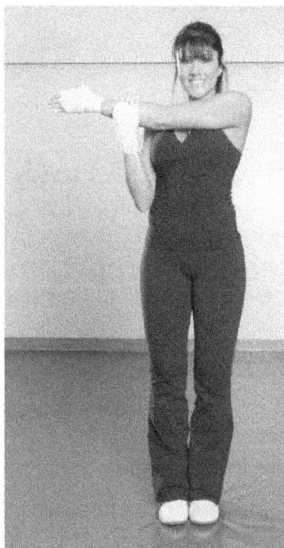

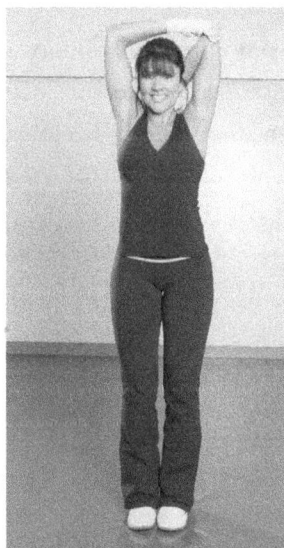

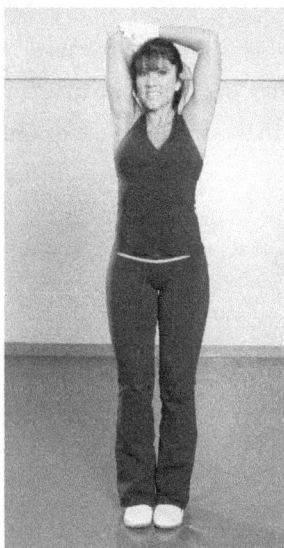

THE MOVE

Stretching is so important. I know that it sometimes seems useless and boring, but it is necessary in order to prevent injury and, believe it or not, for relaxation. Stretching my muscles before a workout enables me to exercise without unnecessary pain because I can really exert myself without fear of getting hurt. It also relaxes me, enabling me to have more endurance. If you are stressed, all of your energy is being used up, and you have nothing left for your workout. In this move, you will stretch your arms.

HOW TO DO IT

Start with your right arm. Bring it up and across your body directly to the left, keeping it straight. Use your left hand to pull the right arm toward your chest as far as you can. Hold it for 10 seconds. Remember to breathe. Switch to the left arm, and use your right hand to hold it back. Hold it for 10 seconds and breathe.

Now stretch out your triceps. Bring your right arm up and over your shoulder, with the elbow bent so that it is pointing toward the ceiling. Your right hand should be touching your right shoulder blade. Use your left hand to grab your elbow and pull it toward your head and behind it, giving your arm a good stretch. Hold this for 10 seconds and breathe. Switch to the left arm, with your right hand holding the elbow. Hold it for 10 seconds and breathe.

Now bring your arms down and go into a march. Simply march in place for 15 seconds, bringing your knees up and swinging your arms to stretch out the tension. Now it's time for round 1!

Round 1

Are you ready to start round 1? Get ready to sweat!

Bob and Weave

THE MOVE

This move is crucial in boxing and is a great workout for the legs and the glutes. When you bob in boxing, you are squatting down to avoid the punch being thrown at your head, and when you come back up, you are going to execute your own punch. So throughout the fight you spend much of your time bobbing and weaving.

Some fighters like myself are not normally bobbers and weavers. Instead, I like to use more lateral movements, where I step to the side to avoid a punch and then come back into the line of fire, so to speak, with my counterattack. But for a workout, the bob and weave is the most effective.

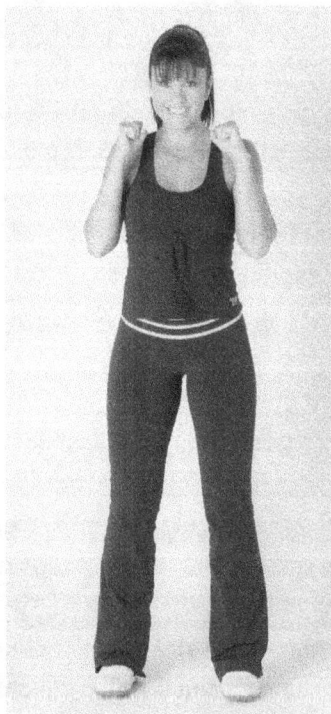

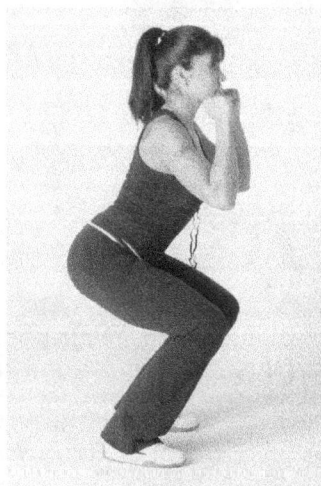

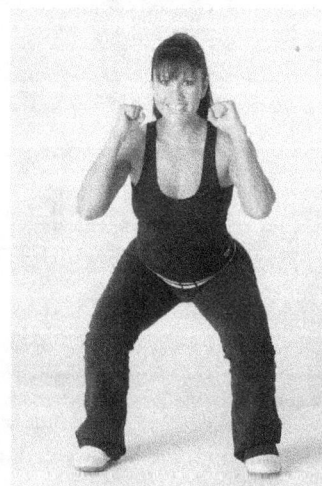

When you weave in boxing, you are going from side to side: you come up with your head slightly to the right, then go back down, then come up with your head slightly to the left. In this workout, though, you can come up with your head straight since no one will actually be throwing punches at you!

HOW TO DO IT

Stand facing forward, with your feet shoulder width apart. I suggest grabbing a pair of 3- to 5-pound weights and holding one in each hand. Squat down as if you are going to sit, keeping your back straight and your chin up. You can hold your hands up by your face, as I like to do, or keep them at your sides.

Squat until your quadriceps are parallel to the floor, then squeeze your glutes as you come back up to the starting position. Do not lock your knees, and be sure to push off with your feet, using your leg strength and not your back. You're going to do this for about 60 seconds. Bring it up and down. It's very simple. This is a great exercise because you are really working your quads at the same time.

Now march in place for 15 seconds.

Jab Punch

THE MOVE

Simply continue with your hip rotations, but this time you will add a punch to the movement. This enables you to get an even better stretch. So you punch to the left, then to the right, as you rotate your hips with each punch.

HOW TO DO IT

Stand facing forward with your feet shoulder width apart. Rotate your hips to the right, extending your left arm out to a punch, without locking the elbow. Your punch should be at chest level. Your right hand is in a fist and remains close to your cheek, with your elbow tucked in at your side.

Turn your back leg with each punch to face the direction of the punch, which gives you the freedom to extend your punch even farther. It actually looks as if you are punching to the side and not directly in front of you.

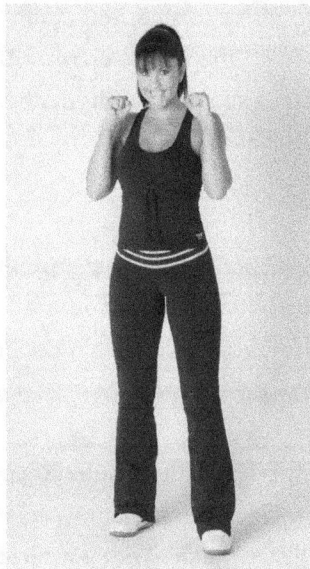

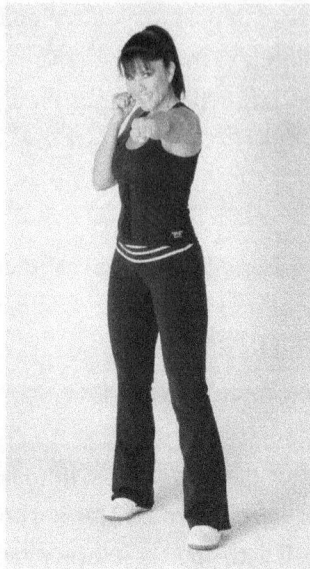

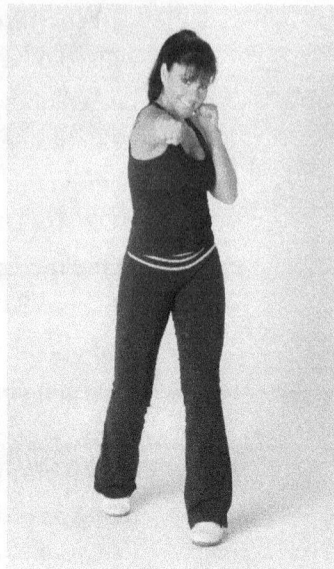

Then throw a punch with the opposite fist: rotate your hips to the left, extending your right arm out to a punch at chest level, without locking the elbow. Your left hand is in a fist and remains close to your cheek, with your elbow tucked in at your side.

Alternate your punches as you rotate your hips with each punch.

Hooks and Uppercuts

THE MOVE

These are two of the most difficult punches in boxing to execute effectively, but don't get discouraged because you are here to get in shape, and for that purpose they are much easier.

First, the hook (see the photos in the top row on page 59): Imagine that you are throwing your fists to punch either side of someone's head. The most commonly thrown punch is the left hook to counter the opponent's jab. Boxers also use hooks to the sides of the opponent's body.

Second, the uppercut (see the photos in the bottom row on page 59): Now imagine throwing your fists directly under someone's chin. It can be a dangerous punch to throw in the ring, but outside of the ring it's awesome because it really works your inner delts. I love to use this punch, especially with weights before a fight. (For more on how to figure out the right size of weights for yourself, see the list in the section called "My Favorite Weight-Training Exercises" in chapter 8.)

HOW TO DO IT

For the hooks: If you are right-handed, stand facing forward in your boxing stance, with your feet shoulder width apart, your left foot in front and your right foot in back. If you are left-handed, simply reverse this stance.

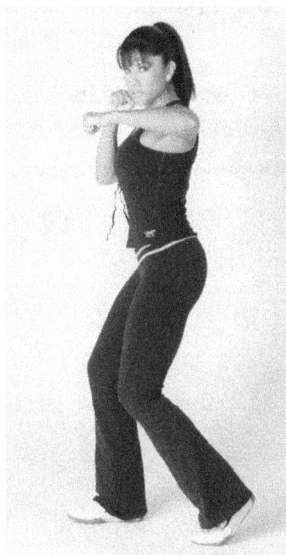

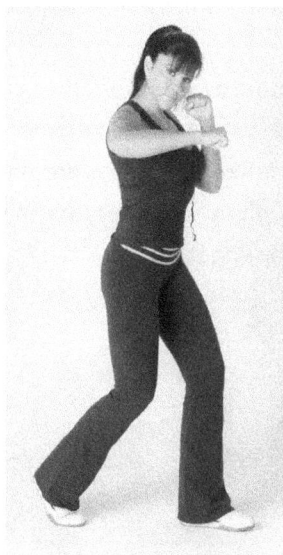

Inhale in this starting position, then turn to the right as you did in the hip rotations, and bring your left hook across your body to the right, so that your left hand and arm with bent elbow come up, over, and across as you exhale. Your leading foot pivots along with the direction of the punch. Your back foot remains pointing forward. Recoil the punch back to the starting position, and inhale. Then rotate your hips to the left, and throw a punch with your right hand, bringing your right fist and arm with bent elbow up, over, and across to the left as you exhale. Your back leg has pivoted slightly to the right in the same direction as the punch.

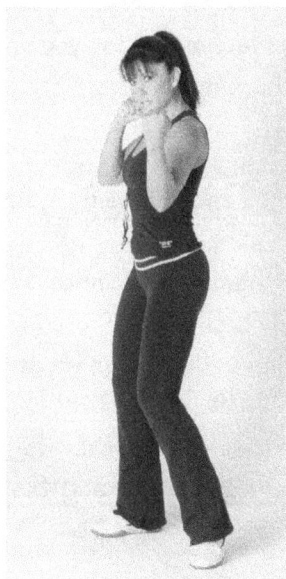

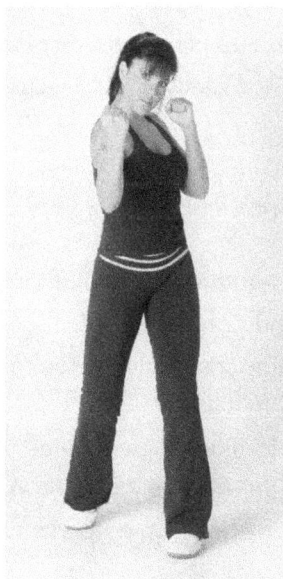

For the uppercuts: Remain in your boxing stance, fists by your cheeks. As before, if you're right-handed, you should stand with your left leg forward; if you're left-handed, stand with your right leg forward. Inhale. Then exhale as you rotate your hips to the left, bend slightly downward, and bring your left fist up as if to land a punch underneath your opponent's chin, while your body follows in the direction of the punch. Be sure you keep the elbow of your punching arm bent. Your feet remain in position. Recoil back to the starting position and inhale. Rotate to the right, bend slightly downward, and as you exhale bring your right fist up with an uppercut underneath the chin of your opponent. For the purposes of getting in shape, imagine that your opponent is taller than you, so that your punch has to extend upward to contact his or her chin. Remember to keep the elbow of your punching arm bent. Recoil back to the starting position and inhale.

Now you'll put all of these moves together. Do a left hook, then a right hook, and a left uppercut, then a right uppercut. Keep alternating punches following this pattern. Be sure to squeeze your abs during this movement and really twist your body, especially with those uppercuts. In boxing, no matter what you're doing, you're always working your abs.

Now that you have it down, do these moves for 60 seconds.

The Speed Round

THE MOVE
This round is done at a high intensity level and a fast pace. I want you to really give it all you've got. You don't have to worry about technique, and you don't have to do it perfectly. You really want to focus on burning calories.

HOW TO DO IT
You will now take all of the punches you have learned and put them together in double time.

Start with the left jab, then the straight right, then your left hook, right hook, left uppercut, and right uppercut. Your body is constantly rotating to the left and the right with each punch. You're going to do this for about 60 seconds.

Next, go into double time—a pace twice as fast as you normally do the move—and just remember to keep your elbows in and punching it out. Keep it going. Punch it out. Then bring it down to a march for 15 seconds.

Leg Stretch

THE MOVE

Now, you're going to stretch your legs. Again, stretching is a very important part of the workout. This is called the straddle stretch.

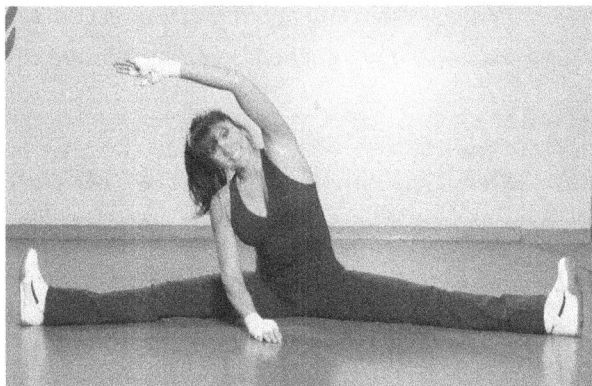

HOW TO DO IT

Sit on the floor with your legs spread out to each side, toes pointing up to the ceiling. Rotate your upper body to the left, and while keeping your back straight, touch your nose to your left knee or as close to it as you can. Hold this position for 30 seconds and remember to inhale and exhale.

Then rotate your body to the right, and touch your nose to your right knee. Hold this pose for 30 seconds and inhale and exhale. Now bring your body to the center and try to touch your nose to the floor, or as close to it as possible, while keeping your back straight. Hold this position for 30 seconds and come back up to the starting position. Get up slowly, and you can start round 2!

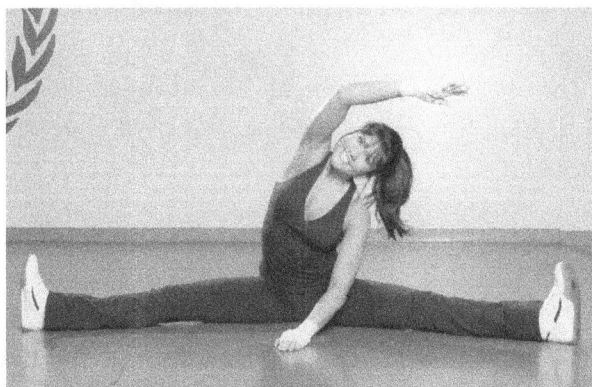

Round 2

Lunges

THE MOVE

In this round, you're going to focus on your legs and butt by doing lunges. The lunges will help tone your leg and glute muscles. I'm addicted to lunges! I have been doing them for years, and I can't think of a better leg workout. The lunge works every part of the leg, as well as the butt.

HOW TO DO IT

Start from a standing position, with your feet facing forward, shoulder width apart. Keep your arms up in the boxing stance with elbows bent. I like my fists right beside my cheeks. You're always thinking about protecting yourself in boxing. Bring your right leg out in front of you, and bend the knee at a 90-degree angle.

As you go down, keep your back nice and straight. Do not let your right knee go forward past your ankle. Your left leg will come down as well. Then push off with your right foot to get back to the starting position. Next, repeat the move with your left leg forward.

This move will help improve your balance. Squeeze your leg muscles as you go up and down. Alternate lunging with your right and left legs forward for a total of 30 repetitions. If you really want to push yourself, hold a light dumbbell in each hand during this exercise. (For more on how to figure out the right size of weights for you, see the list in the section titled "My Favorite Weight-Training Exercises" in chapter 8.)

Bring it down to a march for 15 seconds.

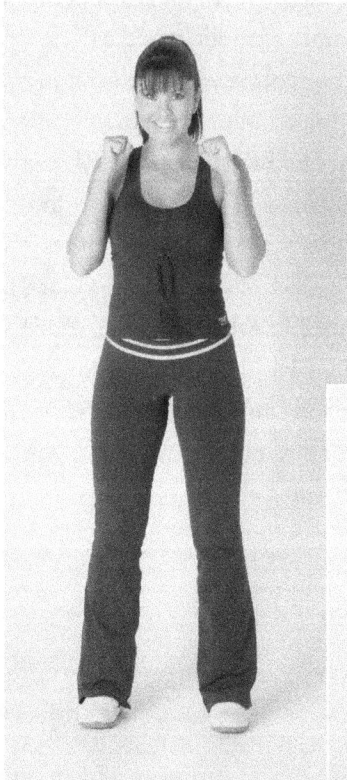

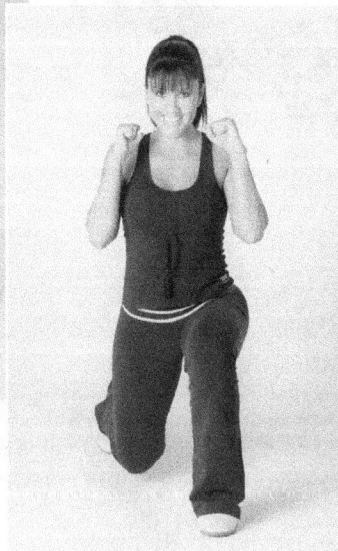

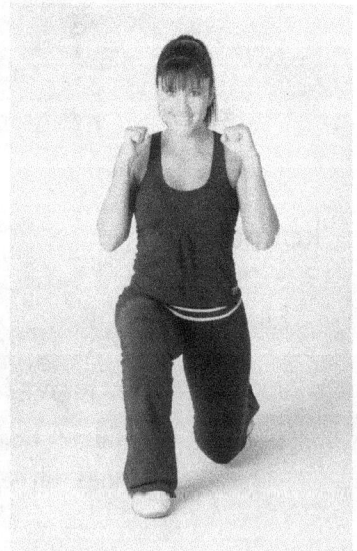

THE MOVE

If you were using weights with the lunges, you can put them down because you are now going to add punches to your lunges. This move is a lunge with a left jab, then a straight right punch. I like this exercise because you are going to hold your position for a bit while you punch, making the move increasingly more difficult.

HOW TO DO IT

Lunge with either foot first and hold the position while you execute a left jab, then a right punch. In boxing, a left jab is called number 1, and a right punch is a number 2. So each time you are in your lunge position, you will throw your 1, 2, and come back up. When lunging, be sure to punch with the opposite hand.

Start from a standing position. Keep your arms up with the elbows bent. I like my fists right by my cheeks. You're always protecting yourself in boxing. Bring your right leg out in front of you, and bend the knee at a 90-degree angle. As you go down, keep your back nice and straight. Don't let the knee go forward past your ankle. The left leg will come down as well, with your knee close to the

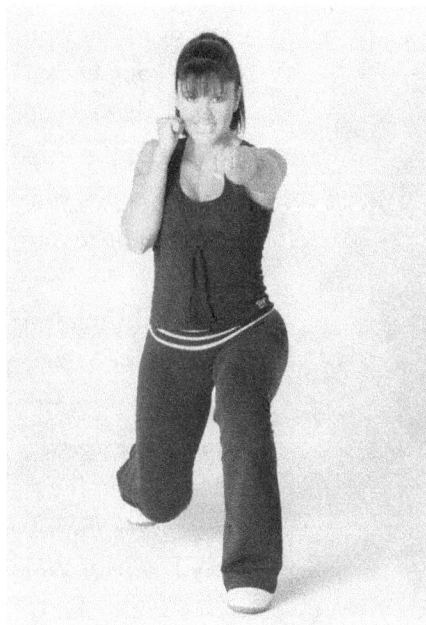

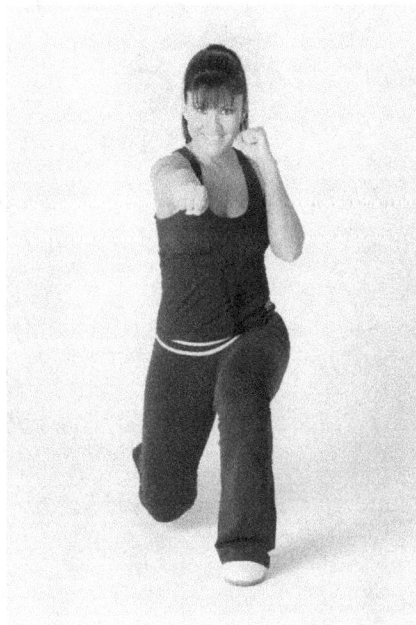

ground. Execute a left jab, then a right punch. Return to a standing position. This move will help improve your balance. Squeeze your leg muscles as you go up and down. Alternate lunging with your right and left legs forward for a total of 30 repetitions.

Bring it down to a march for 15 seconds.

Back Kicks

THE MOVE

I love back kicks because they really work your glutes. Doesn't everyone want a firm, round behind? You sure don't want a flat, sagging one, do you?

I normally do the back kicks while standing, but if you are a beginner, you will start on the floor on your hands and knees. I often used the back kick in Tae Kwon Do competitions, and if you're fast, it works wonders. You essentially have to be fast enough to turn your body backward and execute a kick before you get countered.

In this exercise, instead of snapping your back kick outward, you will simply stretch it outward and upward.

HOW TO DO IT

Get down on your hands and knees. Keep your back straight; try not to arch it. Extend your right leg outward and bend the knee upward at a 90-degree angle, while at the same time really squeeze your glutes. Repeat this 15 times, then switch legs and do 15 reps on the other side. Try for a total of 30 reps for each leg. You may want to use ankle weights after you've gotten used to the exercise. (For more on how to figure out the right size of weights for you, see the list in the section titled "My Favorite Weight-Training Exercises" in chapter 8.)

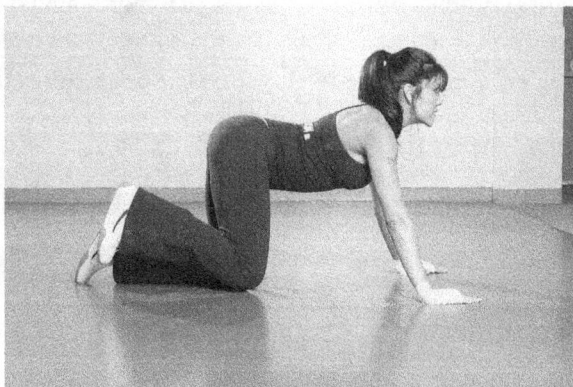

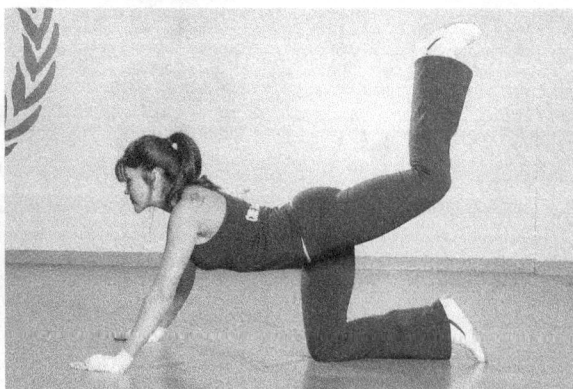

Keep your elbows in and your back nice and flat, and squeeze those glutes. Use nice form, but it doesn't have to be perfect.

Return to a standing position, and bring it down to a march for 15 seconds.

The Speed Round

THE MOVE

You're going to start with my favorite kick in Tae Kwon Do—the front kick. This is an easy move to execute. In a moment, I'll go into more detail on how you can do this move more effectively. For now, let's just get you familiar with the basics.

HOW TO DO IT

Stand with your feet about shoulder width apart and your knees slightly bent. Your upper body is erect, your neck and head are up as you look forward. Hold your arms close to your sides, elbows bent with your fists by your cheeks. Squeeze your abs tight.

Raise your right leg up and in front of you. Bend your knee and bring the right upper leg up and back toward your body. Now kick by extending your right foot directly out in front of you until your right leg is straight. The strike position for the right foot will be the ball of the foot, and your toes will point toward the ceiling. Remember to squeeze your abs as you kick. Then bring the leg back to the starting position.

You're going to do a kick out/bring it back/kick out/bring it back sequence for about 15 seconds and then switch sides. Really kick it out there.

Always remember to breathe. Exhale as you kick forward, and inhale as you bring the leg back. To really kick up the intensity, you can do these double-time (that is, twice as fast).

Bring it down to a march for 15 seconds.

The Quad Stretch

THE MOVE

In the last few exercises you used a lot of your quad muscles, so now you're going to give them a good stretch, especially since you're getting ready to go into your kicking for round 3.

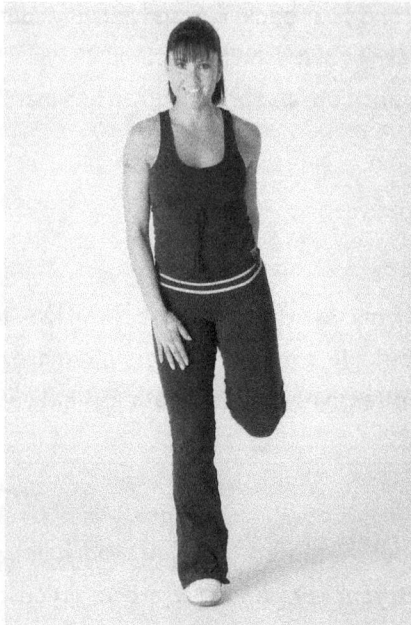

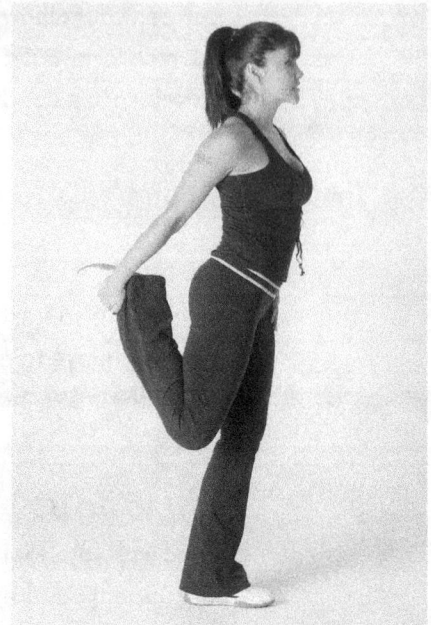

HOW TO DO IT

Stand facing forward, with your feet shoulder width apart and your body upright and erect. Your neck and head are looking forward, and your abs are tight.

Bend your left knee and grab your left foot behind you with your left hand. Pull your foot toward your glute and squeeze. Feel this right in the quadriceps. You can use your other hand to lean against a wall for support if you need to.

You really want to give it a good stretch. Breathe in and out in a controlled manner. Then switch legs. Hold each position for 30 seconds.

Round 3

Front Kick

THE MOVE

In the martial arts this is probably the most basic kick and, in my opinion, the most effective. Not only is it powerful in fighting, but it's a great workout for the quads. It is not a difficult kick to learn, either.

HOW TO DO IT

Stand in your fighting stance again, with your lead foot forward (left or right, whichever is more comfortable); for me, it's my left foot that leads. In the photos below, however, I am leading with my right foot, as well as in the following instructions.

Stand with your right foot forward. Lift your right knee to a 90-degree angle and kick your foot straight out to the front, then bring it back and down to the ground. Your right foot is still in front of your left foot. When you kick outward, you do it in a snapping motion and you recoil rapidly. Switch feet, and now kick with your left leg or your back leg. When that leg comes down, it goes back to the rear position.

Repeat 15 times for each leg. March in place for 30 seconds, and repeat another 15 times per leg. To make this exercise more difficult, when you extend your kick out, hold it for 2 seconds before recoiling and bringing it back down. You should feel it in your quads.

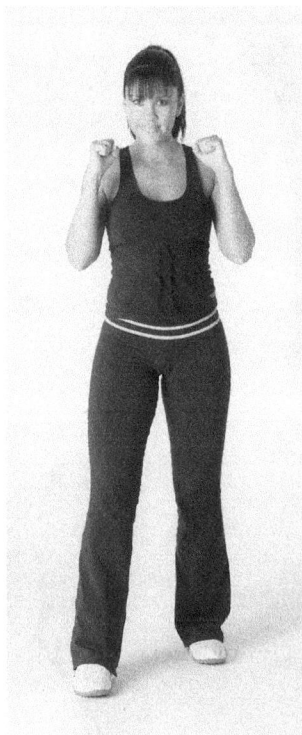

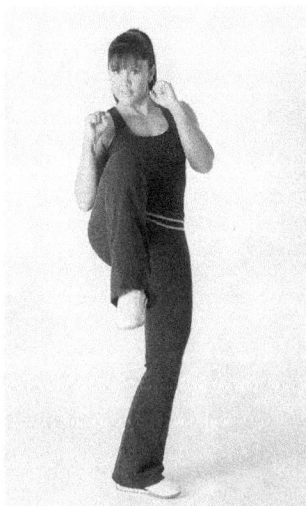

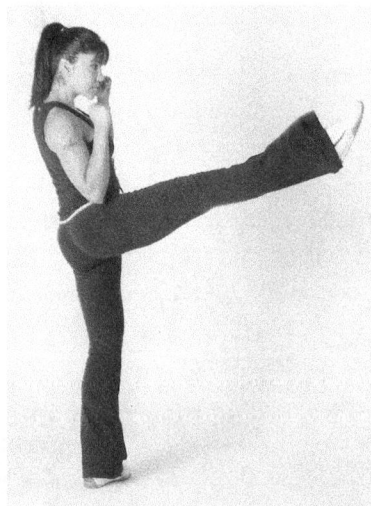

Roundhouse Kick

THE MOVE

This is a more difficult kick, but an absolutely fun one! These kinds of kicks really make Tae Kwon Do an art. The roundhouse is similar to the front kick, only it's done at an angle.

HOW TO DO IT

With your arms in fighting position or your boxing stance, lift your left knee just as you would with a front kick, only this time your knee is pointing to the side or roughly a 90-degree angle. (See a full description of the roundhouse kick in chapter 8.) Now extend your left leg outward in a snapping motion and recoil

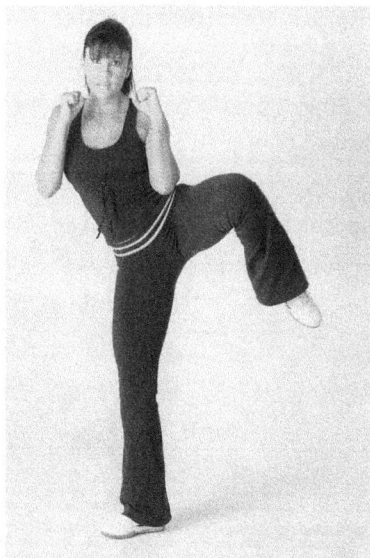

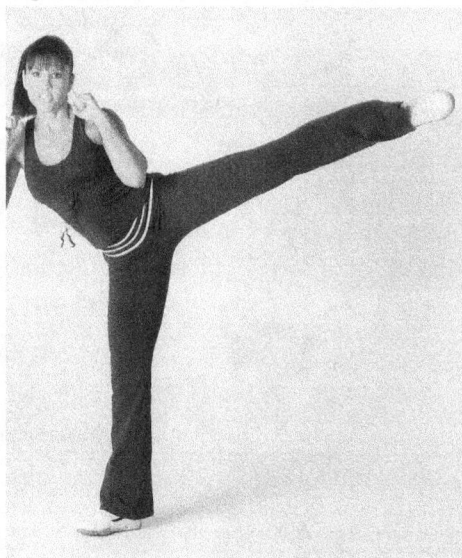

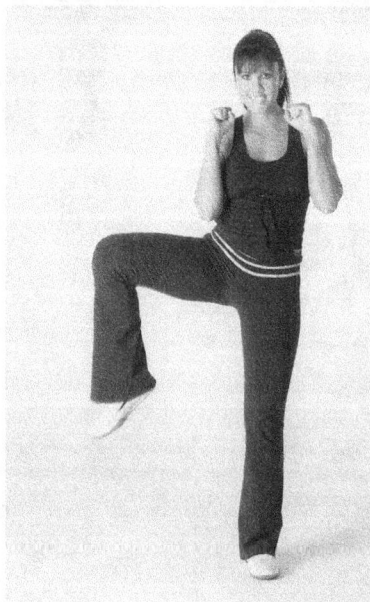

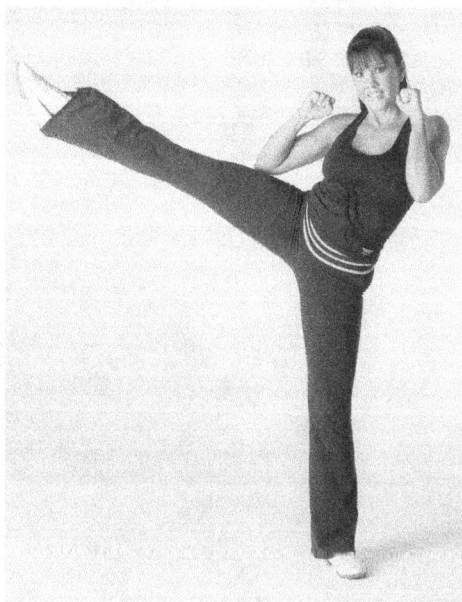

and bring it down to the original position. Repeat this move 15 times, then switch and repeat 15 times with the right leg. Rest a moment, and then repeat 15 more times with each leg.

Squat and Roundhouse Kick

THE MOVE

With your arms in fighting position or your boxing stance, you'll go into a squat and then come up and do a roundhouse kick. This move is the same as the last one, except that you will squat first and then come up with the kick. You'll really feel this in your glutes and quads, and you'll definitely break a sweat, if you haven't already!

HOW TO DO IT

Place your feet about shoulder width apart and turn them slightly out. Put your fists up near your cheeks, as you get into your bob and weave starting position. With a slight arch in your lower back and your head up and looking straight ahead, squat down until your thighs are about parallel to the floor. Always make sure your knees are aligned over your big toes. (See the photos on page 56, for the beginning stance of this exercise, before the kick is executed.) Then come up with a roundhouse kick, and squat back down in the starting position. Kick with alternate legs after each squat.

Squeeze your glutes. Kick it out. Bring these squats down as low as you can, and when you come up, really squeeze your glutes. Repeat for a total of 30 reps. This really burns calories and works the muscles.

Go into your march for 15 to 30 seconds while you breathe deeply.

The Speed Round

THE MOVE
Roundhouse kicks.

HOW TO DO IT
Stand erect in the boxing position, your fists near your face. Instead of bringing your leg down after each roundhouse kick, keep your leg in the air and kick at a higher intensity and a faster pace for 30 seconds on each leg.

Hip Flexor Stretch

THE MOVE

Now, you'll do some stretching, to stretch out the hip flexors. This stretch is vital for me. Especially as I get older, I notice that I need this stretch more and more.

HOW TO DO IT

Get on your knees and put your hands on your hips, with your fingers facing forward and your bent elbows pointing backward. Bring one knee up, with the foot remaining on the floor. Lean forward, pushing your hips forward. Keep your back straight and your head up. You can also place your hands on your front knee as you push forward. Hold this position for 30 seconds and then switch legs.

Stand up and get some water!

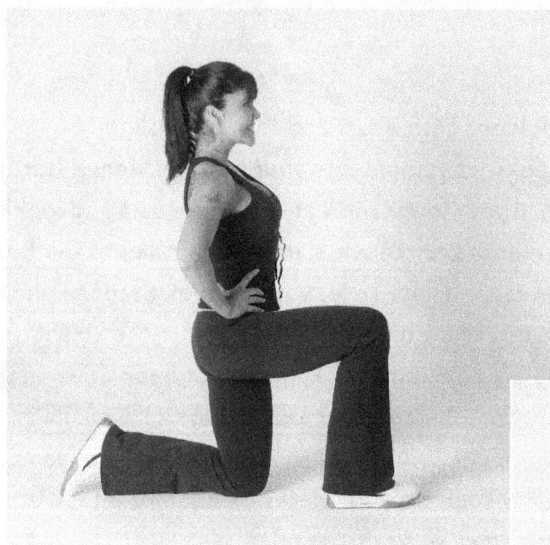

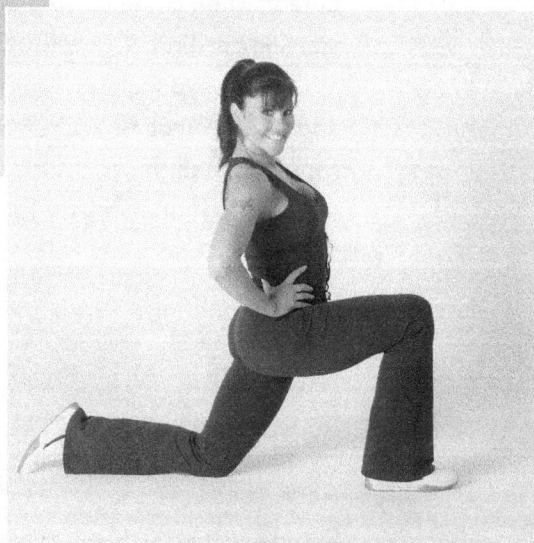

Round 4

THE MOVE

In this round, you're going to work your shoulders. You'll start with the side raise, then do the front raise, and finish with the bent-over rear delt raise. I suggest using dumbbells for shoulder raises. (For more on how to figure out the right size of weights for you, see the list in the section titled "My Favorite Weight-Training Exercises" in chapter 8.) You never want to have that slumped-over look, so building up your shoulders will prevent this. There are three parts to the shoulder, and you will work all three of them.

HOW TO DO IT

The side raise: Stand facing forward with your feet shoulder length apart, and bend slightly forward. Keep your back flat. Raise your arms straight out to the sides, keeping the elbows straight but not locked. Your hands (holding the dumbbells) have the palms facing inward as you start to raise your arms, and when your arms are raised straight out to the sides your palms face the floor. Bring your arms back down to your sides, with your palms facing your sides, and repeat 10 times.

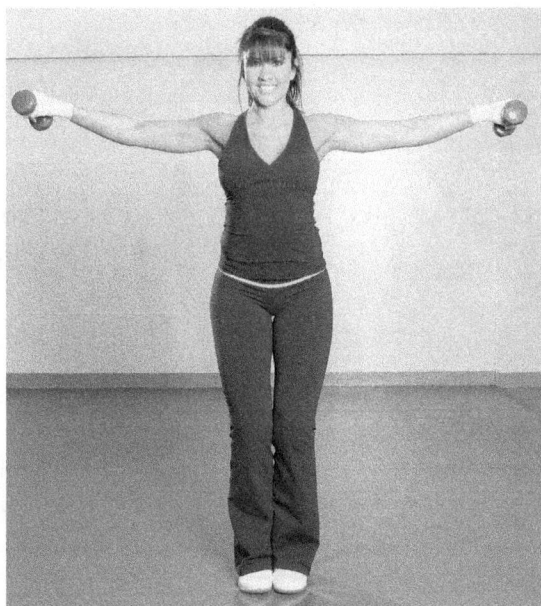

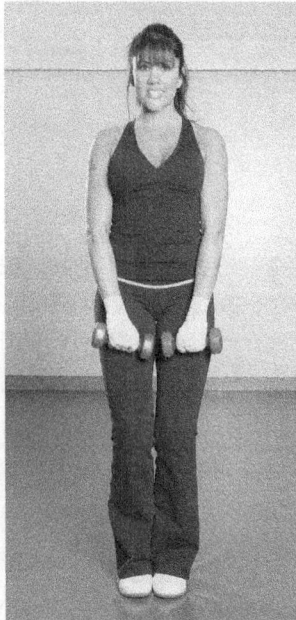

The front raise: Stand up straight, and bring your arms directly in front of you, holding the dumbbells straight down and slightly below hip level, with your palms facing your body. Keeping your arms extended straight out in front of you and parallel to each other, raise your arms up, holding the dumbbells slightly above the level of your head. Keep your arms straight but don't lock your elbows. Repeat this movement 10 times, nice and slow. Hold your arms for a moment at the top, and then slowly bring them down. You can raise your arms faster, but on the way back down, make sure you do it slowly.

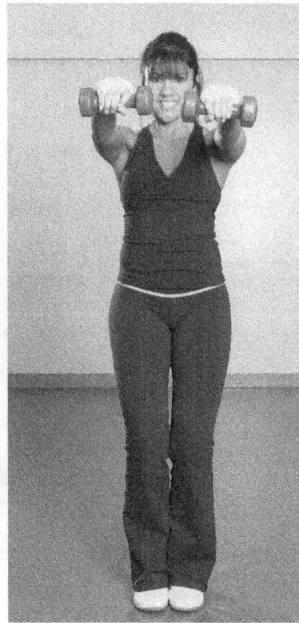

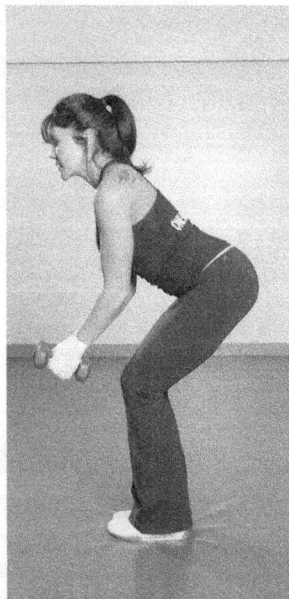

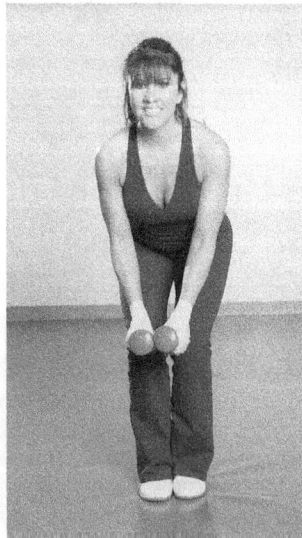

The bent-over rear delt raise: Now you'll switch to the rear delt raise. This exercise will work your rear deltoid muscles. Stand with your feet shoulder-width apart. Squat about halfway down, with your back arched and your buttocks jutting out, and feel the muscles in your thighs and calves as they support you in this position. You are holding the dumbbells in front of you (or to your sides), touching and parallel to each other,

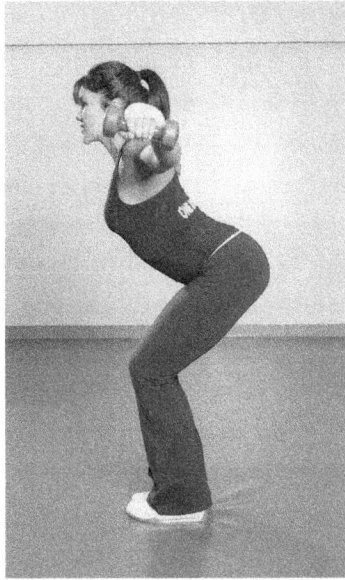

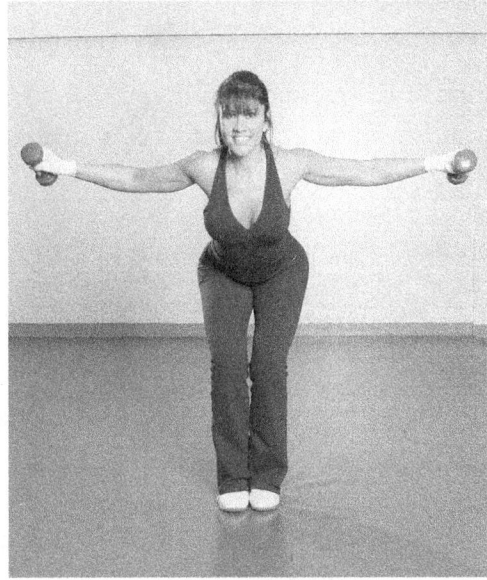

with your elbows slightly bent, your palms facing each other, and your arm and shoulder muscles flexed. Raise your arms up and straight out to the sides, with your palms facing downward, holding the dumbbells. Lift your arms until the dumbbells are at shoulder level. Remember to keep your arms straight, but don't lock your elbows. Then bring your arms down in front of you again, in the same position that you started in (see the photos on page 72, for a front and a side view). Repeat this movement 10 times, fast on the way up and then *slow* on the way down.

Shake your arms out.

Lunge and Front Kick

THE MOVE
Your next move will be starting with the lunge and then coming up with a front kick. This is a great exercise. Don't worry about technique because you really want to concentrate on toning your muscles. You have already learned the lunge and the front kick; now you will put them together. Balance is key in this exercise.

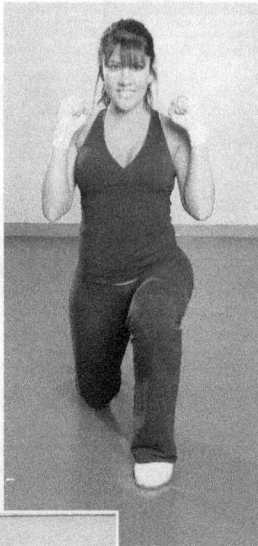

HOW TO DO IT

Put your fists up by your face and keep your elbows in, in boxing stance. You are facing forward, with your feet shoulder width apart. Now lunge forward with your left leg in front, as your right leg bends behind you, the knee almost touching the floor. While you are in the forward position, throw a punch straight in front of you with your right arm. Pull the punch back in, and as you push yourself up with your left leg (which is in front), put your fists back in the boxing stance. Next, bend your right knee and bring the right upper leg up high and back toward your body, then throw it forward straight out into a front kick. Bring your right foot down, and you're back in the starting position. Switch legs, lunging with your right leg in front, and repeat the entire move. Do 10 repetitions on each side.

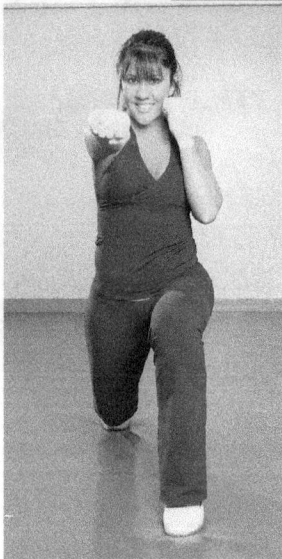

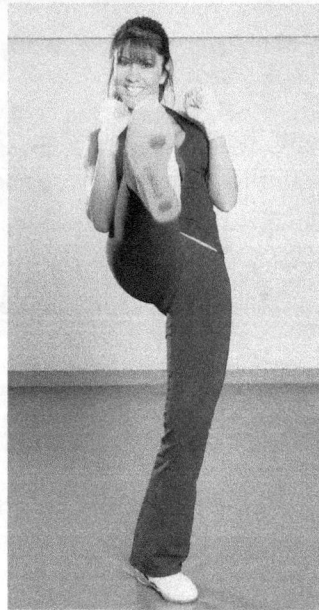

If you bring your kick up as high as you possibly can, you can really feel this in your quads.

Squat and Front Kick

THE MOVE

You have already learned the squat and the roundhouse kick. Now you are going to do the squat with a front kick. The difference is that you will kick to the front instead of to the side, thus working a different set of muscles.

HOW TO DO IT

Squat down in your bob-and-weave starting position, and come up with a front kick using your right leg. Then squat back down in the starting position and come up with a front kick with the left leg. Return to your squat in the starting position, and keep alternating legs as you kick. Refer to the photos below as well as the photos for "Front Kick" (see page 67). Repeat this movement 15 times on each leg.

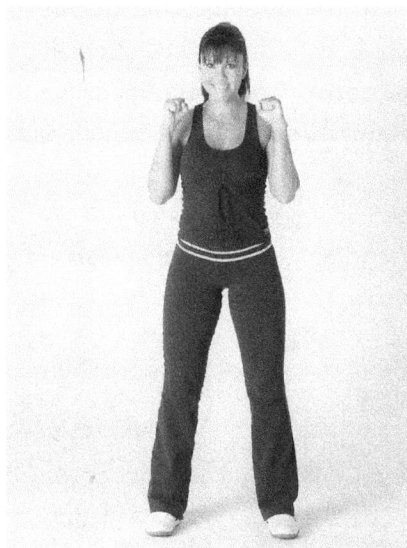

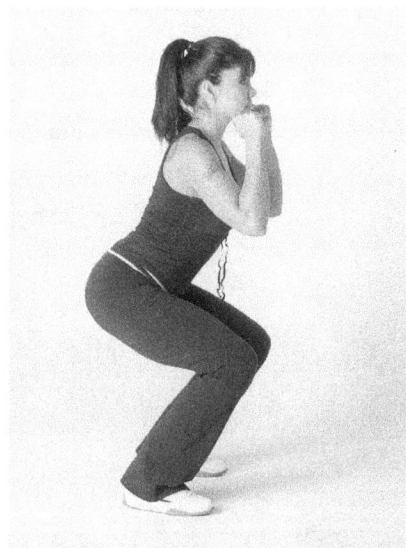

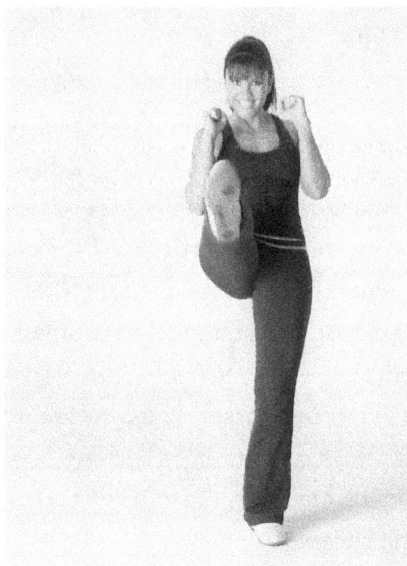

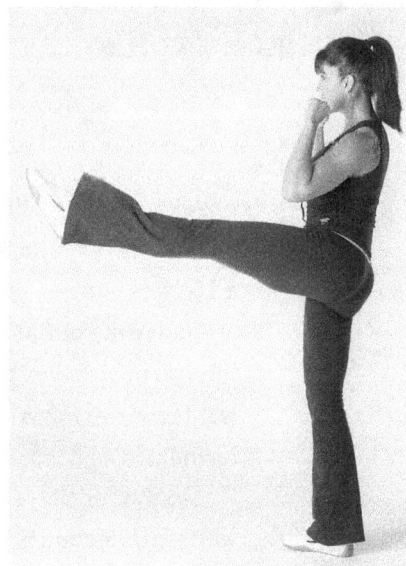

THE MOVE

For this speed round, you're going to do front kicks. This is similar to the speed round you did with the roundhouse kicks, only now you'll do front kicks. Balance will be crucial in this move as well.

HOW TO DO IT

Instead of bringing your leg down after the front kick, keep your upper leg up high and back toward your body with your knee bent, then kick outward and bring it back to this same position, with your upper leg high and knee bent. Keep kicking out for a total of 30 seconds. Switch legs and repeat for another 30 seconds.

Breathe in. Exhale. Take a deep breath. Exhale.

Okay, let's finish your workout with the abdominals.

Crunches with Punches

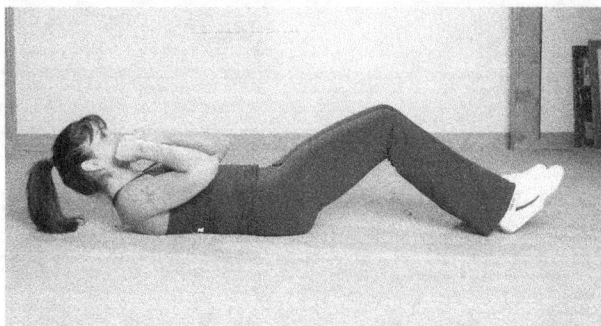

THE MOVE

This exercise will really work your abs until they burn! To do these crunches, you'll lie on a mat or on padded flooring.

HOW TO DO IT

Keep your back nice and flat against the floor, with your fists by your cheeks, elbows in. Bend your legs slightly at the knees as you raise your shoulders off the ground, keeping your neck straight. As you come up, punch with a 1, 2. Remember, that's your left jab, then right punch.

Squeeze your abs as you come up, punch with your left and right fists, and then go back down. Breathe out when you contract. Keep your legs bent. If you want to make this a little easier on yourself, you can extend your legs out a bit farther.

Do this for 50 reps, or you can split it up into two sets of 25 if you need to, with a 30-second break in between.

THE MOVE

In addition to working your legs, this is also a great ab workout.

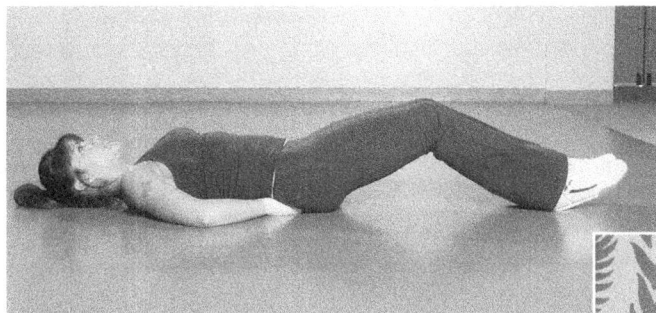

HOW TO DO IT

Lying on your back on the floor, place your hands under your bottom, palms down. Keep your legs nice and straight, bring

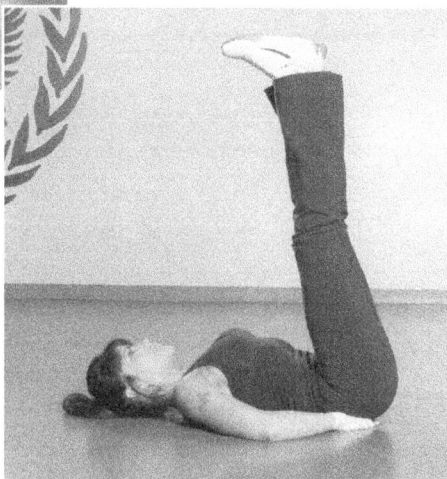

them up to a 90-degree angle, then slowly bring them back down. Repeat the motion 50 times or split it up into 2 sets of 25, with a 30-second break in between.

Keep your abs nice and tight, and remember to exhale on the way back down.

HOW I SEE IT   Intense, but short, running, weight, and bag workouts prepare me for the fast-paced boxing I'll experience in a fight. To be honest, however, if I wasn't making a living as a boxer, I'd skip the short speed work in favor of longer, slower, two or more hour runs.

Call me crazy, but I *love* long-distance running and other types of endurance exercise. If I wasn't training for boxing, I'd run one marathon after another! So, to balance the two, I tend to do my longer, slower workouts during my off season. This allows me to satisfy my craving for distance. As I've learned—and over time you will, too—you must strike a balance between the exercise you *love* and the exercise you *need*, and, if you are lucky, you'll learn to love what you need.

You Did It!

Way to go! You just finished Level One of the Knockout Workout.

You'll be moving on to my favorite weight-training exercises in chapter 8, so get ready for more great results!

5

Knockout Nutrition

I f you do it right, simply eating the proper foods at certain times during the day will make a huge impact on how quickly your body changes.

When I hit forty, after having kids, my weight became difficult to control. Every year it seems harder and harder. If you have kids, chances are you are always on the go. You often wonder when it will ever stop. As for cooking, who has the time?

As you get older, your metabolism slows down. But if you exercise and eat right, you can get in as good a shape as people in their twenties—if not better.

One eating strategy that helped me keep my weight under control was making my lunch the night before and bringing my meal to work the next day. It was a great way to satisfy my stomach (and my brain) and stabilize my blood sugar. This kept me from being tempted by the fast-food places I saw every day. I always carried around healthy snacks for the kids and me, whether in the car, in the gym, at home, or anywhere we went.

For years, many people have mistakenly paid too little attention to nutrition and then assumed that if they worked out long and hard enough, their bodies would radically change. The reality is, that's only partly true, because what you eat significantly impacts how you look and feel. Think about it. If you scarfed down a 500-calorie piece of cake, it would probably bring you about one minute of pleasure. But burning those 500 calories off in the gym (depending on your body weight and exercise intensity level) could take thirty minutes or more of strenuous exercise. Is that a good trade-off? I don't know about you, but my time is too valuable. I've got too many things I'd rather do each day than exercise my butt off in some gym just to burn the fat that resulted from my one-minute indulgence in excess calories that I really didn't want or need.

Proper eating simply means making smart choices that benefit you and will let you reach your goal quickly, and avoiding or cutting down on foods that won't. But if you're exercising properly (that is, getting enough of it, making your muscles work correctly, and so on), you can still eat your favorite foods. Hey, I'm just like you. I love Mexican food and junk food. Would it surprise you to know that I eat dark chocolate and frozen yogurt once a week? And the great thing is, they don't have any negative effects on my body and my appearance. But keep in mind that I work out every day as well.

I'm able to eat like this because most of my diet consists of good, wholesome, nutritious foods. Follow that advice, and you'll be smiling all the way to your new smaller-size clothes. My nutrition plan show-cases real food—the stuff that grows in soil and rots if you don't eat it quickly enough. In this chapter, you will learn about the importance of the following five Knockout food groups:

1. Lean protein (eggs, chicken breast, salmon)
2. Fruits (lower-sugar varieties) and vegetables
3. Healthful root vegetables (sweet potatoes, yams, carrots)
4. Whole grains (slow-cooking oatmeal, whole-grain pasta, whole-grain bread, brown rice, quinoa)
5. Legumes (especially kidney beans and nuts)

My Eating Formula

To eat healthfully, day in and day out, it's infinitely easier if you make it a habit. About thirty days will be all the time that's necessary to do this.

We learn new habits through repetition. The more you keep doing something, the better you get at it, right? So, I want you to make it an enjoyable habit to follow my meal-planning formula, one where you'll never have to stop and ask yourself, "What should I eat for breakfast, lunch, and dinner?"

Feel free to change and modify a few things here and there so that the plan works perfectly for your body and lifestyle; however, always follow the core basics of this program and you'll do just fine.

Hydrate, Hydrate, Hydrate!

Let's talk about water. Your body likes to be fed and watered frequently throughout the day. It responds much better to this type of care, rather than when you miss meals, don't drink enough water, or overload your stomach when you do find the time to eat.

Never let feeling thirsty be your signal to drink a glass of water. It's too late by then because you're already dehydrated. I recommend that you drink at least eight to twelve glasses of water per day. And don't worry, you won't be going to the bathroom all day and you don't need to drink that amount of water all at once. Gradually keep adding more and more water to your diet each day until you reach eight to twelve glasses per day.

> **DID YOU KNOW THAT...** It helps if you drink plenty of water before doing any exercise. Some research has shown that for every 1 percent of weight your body loses from dehydration (loss of water), your peak performance can drop by 10 percent.

Some estimates state that an average person needs roughly 64 ounces of water per day just to maintain normal body function. If you're working out (which, of course, you will be on my Knockout Workout plan), staying active and busy all the time, or the weather is hot, not to mention many other circumstances, your body needs *much more* than 64 ounces.

I'll make it easy for you. Drink enough water to match your body weight. If you weigh 150 pounds, drink 150 ounces per day. No, you shouldn't drink it all at one time. Drink the 150 ounces throughout the entire day, from morning to night.

Here are a few bonuses to drinking more water that you'll thank me for:

- Your body will have all the water it needs.
- Your skin will look better.
- Water helps in fat metabolism (i.e., helps your body burn fat for energy more efficiently).
- Your body won't retain water or get bloated if you drink a lot of water. This *is* what happens, however, when you *don't* drink enough water!
- Your muscles look and perform better. Researchers have found that for every 1 percent drop in fluid in your body (from not getting enough water), there can be a 10 percent decrease in muscle strength.

Lots of Small Meals

Your body also responds well when you eat smaller meals and not those big gut-busters for lunch or dinner—especially late dinners. This means eating about every three hours or so. Don't panic when I say to eat every three hours. I'm talking about grazing and eating small, nutritious meals and snacks.

Here's where supplements can help. I know you're busy, probably too busy to cook all of those meals. McDonald's, Wendy's, Burger King, and all of the other fast-food places would love to see you come in regularly, but there's an easier and more nutritious way to get a quick meal.

Enter the meal-replacement protein shake. Lots of companies sell them, and if you use them correctly, they actually work pretty well. What could be faster than to tear open a packet; pour it into a blender with water, juice, or milk; add a banana or strawberries and maybe a little ice; and put the lid on, press the button, and mix it up? Voilá! You, my friend, now have a tasty, nutritious meal.

That's one way supplements can work for you. The other is taking a good multivitamin-mineral capsule with perhaps an additional antioxidant such as vitamin C. Think of vitamins and minerals as the spark plugs your body's engine needs to metabolize the food you eat in order to promote digestion, breathing, healing, recuperation, and so on.

Granted, if you're eating great fresh foods and in just the right quantities, many people will legitimately question whether you need to use vitamins and minerals, and they have a point. Yet how many people always eat perfectly nutritious meals and snacks? Not very many.

So, give yourself a little cheap insurance and take a multivitamin-mineral supplement at breakfast and another during dinner. You might want to add some vitamin C with that, and don't buy the expensive kind. The late two-time Nobel Prize–winner and noted vitamin C researcher Dr. Linus Pauling was known to say that buying the cheapest kind works just as well. I'll give you more recommendations for supplements later in the book.

Eating Should Be Something You Look Forward To and Enjoy

Let's talk about what to eat. Variety is the key word. Don't be like so many people and eat the same few favorite foods week after week after week. That's boring.

Mix things up. Try new foods, unusual varieties of fruits and vegetables. Give your body exotic taste treats, and see how you feel and respond to those foods. Just as with workouts and training, it does a body good to try different things.

Following are a few suggestions I think you'll like.

Which Should I Eat: Protein, Carbohydrates, or Fat?

How about all of them? But within reason and in the right ratios. Carbohydrates are the fuel that your body uses the fastest. You've heard of glucose, right? Well, your body breaks down the carbohydrates you eat into glucose. Glucose is stored in the muscles and the liver as glycogen, and it's the fuel your body most easily and quickly uses for workouts and other activities.

Here's a fact that many people are unaware of. That amazing body of yours will use the food source that you most often give it as its primary source of energy. For example, if you eat a lot of fat, your body will use more fat for fuel; if it's carbohydrates, then carbohydrates will be turned into glycogen as the fuel source. But fat and carbohydrates are not used equally efficiently or effectively.

Remember earlier when I mentioned getting a balance of nutrients? Too much of one nutrient means there won't be enough room for the others, and too much of the wrong nutrient can really cut into your body's workout and recovery fuel. When you eat carbohydrates, try to get about 50 percent from fast-burning simple sugars such as fruit, juices, honey, and so forth, and the other 50 percent from slow-burning complex carbs such as vegetables, beans, grains, pasta, legumes, brown rice, and so on.

Let's Talk about Protein

Working out increases your body's need for nutrients, and if you're doing intense workouts, you'll need more protein than someone who's not as active as you. Try to get between 0.7 and 1.3 grams of protein per pound of your body weight each day.

I'm amazed at how many people still believe the myth that the body can use only 20 to 50 grams of protein at a time. Scientists and researchers I've talked to say they have yet to see a conclusive study that proves this. This means that your body type, age, metabolism, genetics, and activity and intensity levels determine how much protein your body will need at any given time, so experiment and find what's best for you.

Of all the nutrients you eat, carbohydrates are protein sparing. This means that your body will use carbohydrates as its primary fuel before tapping into its protein reserves. And that's what you want to happen because then your body can use more protein for tissue repair and recovery. Aim to get your protein from lean meat, skinless chicken and turkey, fish, egg whites, nonfat dairy products, and skim milk powder.

Those Things Called Electrolytes

Your body loses electrolytes quickly whenever you're physically active. Some quick and easy ways to replace electrolytes can be either drinking a sports drink or eating foods that are probably already in your diet. For example, to replace sodium and chloride, add a little extra salt to your food. To replace potassium, have some fruit, such as oranges and bananas.

Pre-Workout Fuel

One size doesn't fit all if you are deciding what to eat and not eat before you exercise. Some folks believe that eating a meal loaded with complex carbohydrates (such as pasta) the night before you train loads the body with plenty of energy for the next day.

Many others say that having the meal roughly two or so hours before your activity is what makes the difference. Personally, I've found it to be a combination of the two, plus two other variables: the amount of activity I've performed the week before and the overall composition of my diet for that week.

Interestingly, I've found that if I worked out and was physically active for at least three or four days that week, the normal and extra amounts of calories ingested during my meals seemed to have primarily been used for recuperation, repair, and growth after the previous exercise I put my body through, with little left over for additional physical demands.

Yet on the weeks when I did less intense workouts in the gym, outdoors, or in supplemental training and kept my complex carbohydrate intake at 50 percent, protein at 35 percent, and fat at 15 percent, I found that my body had plenty of energy and endurance for whatever activity or sport I was doing.

Just keep in mind that you, I, and everyone else will respond differently to how our bodies use foods and to the various amounts of carbohydrates, proteins, and fats in our diets.

Nutrition Tips

- Try to eat small meals throughout the day, about three to four hours apart.
- Small meals won't overtax your body's ability to digest and assimilate the nutrients and will allow it to better use those nutrients with minimal waste. Small meals keep your blood-sugar levels stable all day and give your body the proper ratio of nutrients it needs when it needs them and in amounts it can optimally use.
- Eat clean to be lean. For the most part, a leaner athlete (within reason) can be a more effective athlete. Excess body fat slows you down; fat takes up space and is not living tissue, as muscle is.
- Lean muscle tissue is living tissue (it needs to be fed with nutrients), and the more muscle you have—within reason—the more of those nutritious foods you can eat. Frequent smaller meals, along with the extra calories your lean tissue needs, help create a metabolic boost that enables your body to burn calories and body fat more efficiently. It's sort of the best of both worlds: eat more calories, lose more fat.
- Always keep in mind, however, that the numero uno factor in losing body fat is the total amount of calories you eat in a day versus the total number of calories you burn in a day.
- Don't be overly concerned about whether you're eating the correct ratio of nutrients, eating them at the right time, and so on. The bottom line is, if you're eating more food than you can use, you're going to get fat.
- Always have a good breakfast, and never miss this meal.
- Choose a different kind of breakfast every day.
- Always drink a glass of water on waking and about twenty to thirty minutes before a meal so that it won't interfere with your digestion.

- During the meal, sip only enough water to help you swallow the food. Drinking too much water with the meal tends to dilute essential stomach acids that are needed to break down nutrients in the food.

Some great breakfast choices include:

- Cottage cheese (nonfat or low fat) and fruit
- Yogurt mixed with muesli, bran, or high-fiber cereal
- Eggs with grapefruit and unbuttered whole-grain bread
- High-fiber, low-fat cereal with skim milk
- Fresh juice with a bagel
- Oatmeal, mixed and cooked with skim milk, honey, and sliced banana and fortified with extra skim milk powder

Some great lunch choices include:

- Dark green salad with tuna (in spring water), turkey or chicken, and a piece of fruit
- Tuna or egg-white salad (made with nonfat mayo, sweet relish, chili powder, celery salt, celery) with nonfat or low-fat whole-grain crackers, a piece of fruit
- Bagel with low-fat chicken or tuna salad spread and a piece of fruit

Some great dinner choices include:

- Fish, lean beef, skinless chicken or turkey
- Pasta (with red sauce, low-fat white sauce, or plain)
- Dark green leafy and fibrous vegetables
- White fibrous vegetables (cauliflower)
- Richly colored vegetables (tomatoes, squash, peppers, and so on)

Some great snack choices include:

- Fruit
- Celery, carrots
- Popcorn (no butter)
- Bagels

- Rice cakes with applesauce
- Turkey jerky

Eating after Your Workouts

I'd like to mention a very important time for you to refuel your body. So important, in fact, that many fitness experts and researchers believe it may be one of the most important meals of the day. It's right after you work out.

Some studies have shown that the body will store more muscle fuel (glycogen) nearly *twice as effectively* in a brief period right after exercise (within about forty minutes) than at other times during the day when you did not exercise. Have a 12-ounce can of fruit juice, and you'll be covered. You might want to dilute the fruit juice with water, as many athletes say this has helped their bodies make better use of the carbs. Try it and see.

My Daily Meal Choices

Over the years, many people have asked me what I typically eat each day for my meals and snacks. Here they are:

Breakfast: Eggs (scrambled plain or with greens or veggies) with a whole grain (oatmeal or bread) or my Whole-Grain Protein Pancakes. See chapter 9 for my pancake recipe.

Lunch: A huge salad (enough to fill a dinner plate) with dark leafy greens, broccoli, beans, raisins, nuts, and lean chicken or fish. Consult my salad recipes in chapter 9 for inspiration.

Dinner: Baked lean protein (salmon or chicken) with a green vegetable (broccoli or spinach), and a whole grain or a healthful tuber (brown rice, yam, quinoa).

Snacks: Depending on your hunger levels, I recommend up to two snacks a day. Make sure your snack contains protein and/or some healthful fat or fiber to slow your digestion and satisfy your hunger. My favorite snacks include a handful of walnuts with a piece of low-fat cheese, one small apple with a handful of walnuts, one small apple with a slice of low-fat cheese, and nonfat yogurt with granola.

My Lean Body Extras

Let me give you some tips that'll really help you keep the extra pounds off and your metabolism fired up.

The Step Forward/Step Back Principle

Are you looking for an incredibly easy way to burn fat, be leaner, have more energy, and yet will allow you to eat more food? You've found it! Thinking like a boxer, I'm calling it Step Forward/Step Back.

You might ask, "Step Forward/Step Back, what the heck is that?" It's simply changing the amount and the kind of food you eat each day. One day you eat more; the next day you eat less. Nothing could be easier or more effective.

You see, your body becomes stagnant—meaning it simply wants to stay right where it is, in its present condition—if you always eat the same foods in the same proportions at the same time each day.

This process of keeping your body's weight and metabolism at the same level is called homeostasis. For your purposes, just remember that once your body gets used to doing the same thing over and over, it doesn't want to change and will fight you tooth and nail to avoid it. That is, unless know how to Step Forward/Step Back.

You've no doubt felt the effects of homeostasis; your body weight tends to stay the same, and it's hard for you to make any lasting changes—either up or down—in your body weight number or in your appearance. That's why so many people resort to drastic measures out of frustration to change how much they weigh. And therein lies the problem; all they seem to care about is losing weight, rather than losing only fat. I could show you how to lose lots of weight in a hurry—how about five pounds in forty-eight hours?—but you would be losing only water weight, not fat.

Try to get this "I want to lose weight" idea out of your mind, because simply focusing on losing weight and attaining some magical weight number will not solve your problem or quench your desire to have a new body, look good, feel great, and have lots more energy.

The majority of people who lose weight end up losing very little fat and lots of lean muscle tissue. This is a major mistake. Fat just sits there and takes up space on your body. It slows you down, keeps you sluggish, and makes you look like someone you'd rather not be.

What you want is lean muscle tissue. Muscle is living tissue, meaning it needs food every day to survive. With fat, it's a different story. And because muscle is living tissue, you can eat more—you've got to feed that muscle—and you'll weigh less, because lean muscle tissue creates a metabolic response that causes your body to burn fat. It really fires up the energy furnace inside your body.

Did you hear that? The more muscle you have, the more you can eat and the more it makes your body burn fat. That is, as long as you're giving your body the right kinds of protein, carbohydrates, and fat that it needs, in the right proportions, throughout the day.

Let me paint a vivid picture for you. Let's say you're a person who weighs 145 pounds and you want to keep all of the muscle you can but want to lose the fat. Let's say your friend is the same height and weighs 145 pounds, just like you; however, all that your friend cares about is *losing weight* and getting down to a certain weight number.

After you work out for a few weeks, using the tips in the Knockout Workout, while your friend has been on the latest weight-loss drug or starving herself as she always has, you both stand in front of a mirror. Get ready because you are about to experience one of the biggest surprises of your lives.

You look at your body, and it's lean and firm and has a great shape. You look at your friend's body and you can't believe what you see: it's flabby, it jiggles, it wiggles, and it looks totally different from yours. But, you ask, how can that be, especially when you both weigh 145 pounds? The difference is in the composition of your bodies and not in how much you weigh. You see, your friend focused on reaching a number and didn't care about eating or exercising correctly. This caused her metabolism to slow down because the drugs or the severely limited food intake curbed her appetite, which resulted in her not eating enough protein, carbohydrates, and fat (in the right proportions) to maintain her lean muscle tissue and keep that metabolic fire burning.

And because she didn't eat enough protein, although her body still needed it, where do you think her body got it from? Her muscles—yes, from lean tissue. Why? Because muscle is made up of protein. In other words, her body fed upon itself (on her lean muscles) so that it could get the nutrients it needed when it needed them. When that happened, the muscle was replaced with fat. If your friend only knew the simple nutritional and exercise tips you're learning, she'd be able to get the results she so desperately wants, without using drugs, diets, and other gimmicks.

Keeping your muscle is very important. Remember, the more muscle you have, the more you can eat, because your metabolism—the furnace inside you that burns food—is burning hot. Muscle is living tissue and needs food, and it keeps your furnace going strong. When your body gets the right balance of proteins, carbohydrates, and fat, the furnace starts to burn your fat, rather than protein from your muscle tissue or those protein-saving nutrients such as carbohydrates.

Talk about a great new look! Your body appears lean and firm because you gave it the nutrients (proteins, carbohydrates, and fats) it needed throughout the day, in the right ratio that it needed them, thereby keeping your food furnace hot and burning fat all day long. The end result is that you can weigh the same as your friend, but you will look 100 percent better because you're leaner and have more muscle. The real you has finally come out of hiding.

Right here and right now, I want you to do one thing: throw out your scale or at least put it away for a while. The scale can be a saboteur to your nutritional and fitness goals. If you live by the scale, you'll always be frustrated by the scale. What most scales never tell you is how you actually look and what the composition of your body is. That is, how much of your weight is fat and how much is muscle. So, put the scale away and let the mirror and your clothes be your guides.

Are You Ready to Step Forward/Step Back?

Now you know that the goal is to keep your muscle and lose excess fat. And you have learned that eating the right portions of protein, carbs, and fat is an important way to do that. But I'm about to reveal something incredible to you.

One of the strangest tricks to help you lose fat and weight whenever you want to, while preserving your lean muscle tissue, is to keep your body off balance by never allowing your body to get used to one thing. You always want to keep it guessing about what the heck you're going to do next.

Oddly enough, this surprise attack actually helps keep your body in balance! Did you get that? Throw it off balance to keep it in balance. And when it comes to eating, Step Forward/Step Back is one of the best ways to do it. Here's how:

1. For seven days, write down what you eat each day. Simply take a piece of paper and write down the kinds of food and the quantities you have eaten—for all meals, including snacks—during that day.

2. Once you have done this for seven days, go to any local bookstore and pick up a book of food counts. This is a book that lists nearly every food and gives you the breakdown of calories, fat, protein, carbohydrates, and so on, for those foods. I highly recommend *The Book of Food Counts* by Corinne Netzer.

3. With your food count book in hand, get out your seven-day list of foods that you've eaten and write down the number of calo-

ries for each food. For example, let's say you had a 5-ounce piece of chicken breast. You'd simply look up chicken in the book, guesstimate the approximate serving size that you had, find the total number of calories for that portion of chicken breast, and you will probably see a number like "140 calories." Then write down "140 calories," and do the same thing for every food you ate during that day and for the rest of the week. This book makes it easy to figure out the calorie counts, and it will take only about fifteen minutes for you to do your complete list, so bear with me. These will be the best fifteen minutes you've ever spent on yourself.

4. After you've found the number of calories for all of the foods you've eaten for each of the seven days, add up the numbers for all seven days to get your total number of calories consumed for the week. For example, let's say your seven-day total comes to 21,000 calories. That's 3,000 calories a day × 7 days = 21,000 calories.

5. Now you have the two numbers you need to start Step Forward/Step Back: the daily average total (3,000 calories) and the weekly total (21,000 calories).

6. Using our 3,000 calorie per day example, here's how you'll Step Forward/Step Back:

> Day 1: eat 2,700 calories
>
> Day 2: eat 3,300 calories
>
> Day 3: cat 2,000 calorics
>
> Day 4: eat 4,000 calories
>
> Day 5: eat 3,500 calories
>
> Day 6: eat 2,500 calories
>
> Day 7: eat 3,000 calories

Do you see what you were doing? You simply changed how much food you ate each day. You never ate the same amount of food two days in a row. Some days, it seems like you're eating a lot of calories, doesn't it? Yet take a good look at the total number of calories you've eaten for the seven days. It's the same 21,000 calories that you were eating before! You didn't eat a single calorie more than in the past, but it's how you ate those calories that caused positive changes in your body. You shocked your body and threw it off balance because you constantly changed how much food you fed it each day. You never gave your body a chance to adapt to what you were doing. This is so easy, yet so powerfully effective.

Do you know what else happened? You also caused your body's food furnace to burn even hotter, thereby helping your body burn more fat more effectively. You did that just by changing how much you ate every day, and you didn't even have to run or go to the gym to do it. Now that's pretty cool.

Here's how Step Forward/Step Back works: Because you eat more calories one day and fewer the next, you throw your body off-balance; it doesn't know how many calories it will get for the next meal, let alone the next day. When that happens, to overcompensate for this surprise, your body's metabolism—the furnace that burns food—becomes faster and hotter, thereby allowing you to burn more calories, eat more food, burn fat, and do it faster than ever before while using the food you ate more efficiently.

Best of all, you are doing it naturally, without drugs or dieting, and even without exercise! If you want super-incredible results in a hurry, however, I'll give you a few quick and effective ways to change your body in a snap. Just stay tuned.

Step Forward/Step Back works great when you vary not only the quantity of food you eat each day, but also the kinds of food eaten at each meal. Always change what you eat, when you eat, and how much you eat, each and every day. Make this a rule for life.

And if you want to lose the fat even faster, slowly reduce your caloric intake each week. Most people make the mistake of changing too many things too quickly, thus they never really know which factor was responsible for their fat loss. Was it the 50 calories a day they cut out? Was it more exercise? Was it more protein and less carbs? Unless you slowly adjust one variable at a time and give it enough time to see how it works, you'll never know what your body responds best to.

That's why reducing calories little by little works so well for people. By keeping their activity levels and everything else in their lives the same, when they change only one variable at a time—such as reducing the amount of food they eat each day by 50 or so calories—they have precise control over what that 50-calorie reduction does or does not do to their bodies.

Once you find the perfect daily and weekly amount of calories for your body, then it's a breeze to pick another variable—like exercise—and change it a bit to see how that affects you. The thing to remember is to take it slow and allow your body enough time to adjust to any change and give you accurate feedback.

As a good rule of thumb, try to eat your biggest meal in the morning or very early in the day and gradually reduce the amount of food you eat during each meal as the day goes on. If you can't manage to eat a hearty breakfast, then have your biggest meal as early in the day as possible.

Many people discover that their metabolism runs faster during the early part of the day. Thus, their bodies are quite forgiving and will more effectively burn any excess calories they eat, if they have them early enough in the day. Bottom line: unless you've got a race-horse's metabolism, stay away from late-night gut-buster meals!

Here's an important thing to remember: when deciding how much food you should eat at a meal, always try to base the amount on what your activity level will be for the next two to three hours. Don't base it on how active you've just been, before the meal. Most people make the mistake of doing the latter.

For example, if you are planning some physical activity like a workout, a walk, or a run, then you should eat more and have more calories about an hour or so before the activity than you would normally eat *after* that workout or physical activity. This way, you'll have plenty of fuel for that activity. So, eat more before you're active and less after the activity is finished.

Another thing Step Forward/Step Back works incredibly well for is PMS (premenstrual syndrome). During those trying days, many women crave all kinds of foods and in quantities they usually don't desire during the rest of the month. If this describes you, that's okay. Go ahead and give your body whatever it craves, whenever it craves it.

You heard me correctly: it's normal and natural. Just don't do it for more than a few days in a row. I'll tell you a little secret: dark chocolate usually makes many women feel better during this time. Just try to avoid binge eating. It can be habit forming, and it won't make you feel any better, only worse.

You'll want to continue experiencing those great results from the Step Forward/Step Back technique, and you can if you simply adjust your eating schedule to reflect those extra calories and cravings. Count the meals and the days you eat more as your high-calorie days in the Step Forward/Step Back schedule. Then in a day or so, when your body has fewer cravings, lower your food intake. These will be the low-calorie days in the Step Forward/Step Back schedule. By simply adjusting your high- and low-calorie days, you will still be eating the same number of calories for the week. Just make sure you don't go over that weekly total number. If you're using 21,000 calories for the week, you always want to stay at the number or slightly below it.

Besides the incredible results you'll experience from using Step Forward/Step Back, another advantage is that before you know it, you won't have to keep count of your foods anymore. You'll soon be amazed at how fast your mind and body will instinctively know just how much or how little you should eat at any given meal. Like a finely tuned machine, your body will tell you when to eat, what to eat, and when to stop. Your body's been trying to talk to you all these years. Now, you're ready to listen.

Finally, I want you to do both of us a big favor: start treating yourself better and don't be so hard on yourself. For heaven's sake, be your own best friend. Whenever you crave certain foods, there's no need to freak out (to either stop eating or do hours of cardio workouts) or do something drastic. Just give your body whatever it wants when it wants it and adjust your intake, eating either less or more food the next day. If you ate a lot today, then don't eat as much tomorrow. It's so simple. In the end, it'll all balance out, and Step Forward/Step Back will always keep you on target.

The Step Forward/Step Back Bonus: Keeping on Track When You Can't Keep Count

Sometimes you may travel or take vacations and leave your comfort zone: the daily activities and everything you normally have access to, such as a gym, certain foods, or a kitchen to cook them in. When people are away from home, it often throws their diets off the tracks. Yet this doesn't have to happen to you, if you follow a few simple tips and guidelines:

1. **Remember to keep it clean and lean.** The less processed and coated your foods are, the healthier they will be and the leaner your body will remain. So whenever you eat out, focus mainly on baked, broiled, steamed, and raw foods.

2. **Make most of the animal proteins you choose lighter in color and fewer of them redder.** In other words, try to get most of your protein from chicken, turkey, eggs, lean dairy, and fish, with fewer of your proteins coming from lean pork loin and beef. The key is to eat something each week from all of the protein groups, but eat more proteins from creatures that swim or fly and less from the four-legged kind that roam the land.

3. **Make sure there's a balance between the last meal and the next meal.** Sometimes when you dine out, the healthy food choices on the menu are very limited. Besides, that famous restaurant's gourmet dishes may taste utterly delicious! Go ahead and enjoy them. Just make sure that your next meal balances out that high-calorie meal. You can easily do this by having a highly nutritious meal that's low in calories and fat, in a smaller quantity than you'd normally eat. When you indulge in a Step Forward meal with a lot of calories, follow it with a Step Back meal that has

many fewer calories. And since you are using a week's food intake as your overall allotment, it's never a problem if you take a nutritional detour for one meal.

4. **Quickly get back in balance by increasing your activity level.** At times you'll want to get back on track with your next meal to balance out what you ate at the previous meal, but you can't because your schedule doesn't allow it or the available food choices prevent this. Don't get upset about it; simply adjust the other important component of your plan and increase the calories your body burns by stepping up your activity level. Walk faster. Walk longer. Take bigger steps and strides. Use the stairs and not the elevator. Park farther away. Make multiple walking trips to get your baggage, groceries, packages, or whatever else you're doing. Anything that makes you move more, breathe more heavily, and be active longer will help offset the effects of what you eat and allow you to keep everything under control.

Powerful Eating Strategies for a Knockout Body

So many times, people think they have to make huge lifestyle and diet changes to see any results. But it's not true! It's so much easier than that. If you follow a few simple rules, I know you'll be very pleased at the changes you'll see and feel.

Don't Eat at Night after You Finish Dinner

A major mistake people make is eating a big dinner late in the evening or having high-calorie snacks too close to bedtime. I've found that in the evening, my metabolism tends to slow down. My body can digest and use a meal's nutrients more effectively earlier in the day than it can metabolize that same meal later at night. For many people who burn fewer calories later in the day, a large late meal or snack may be more easily stored as fat. I suggest that if you're able to have your evening meal before 7:00 p.m. and your bedtime is about 11:00 p.m., eating a light, nutritious protein snack around 9:00 p.m. would be fine.

Always Stop Eating before You Feel Full

We are forever in a hurry, especially when eating our meals. This is a terrible habit. Not long ago, I read that the average person takes less than twelve minutes to eat a meal. We'd probably be healthier if we followed the example of Europeans and certain nationalities who believe that savoring a good meal is one of the joys of life. In many countries, a meal with family and friends can last two or more hours. Although you may not be able to carve two hours out of your busy day for one meal, you can take a little longer to eat and enjoy your food.

Many people don't realize that because they eat such large quantities and finish their meals so quickly, they haven't given their bodies enough time for the stomach to signal the brain, saying that it's full. I tell people to figure it will take about twenty minutes for this to happen.

Here's a good rule of thumb: If you don't have at least twenty minutes to eat slowly, eat wisely, and enjoy your meal, then push yourself away from the table *before* you feel full. (By the way, that's another great triceps exercise for you to do!) Always leave the table feeling a little hungry, as if you could've eaten more. Doing so will keep your calorie intake lower and help you lose fat and excess pounds more quickly. As a result, you will look and feel great.

> **DID YOU KNOW THAT...** There's a simple trick to raise the good cholesterol (HDL) in your body. Do at least ten minutes daily of an aerobic activity such as walking, biking, or any other exercise that gets your heart and lungs pumping.

Drink Water with Meals

I previously mentioned the importance of hydrating your body and giving it plenty of water throughout the day. So, when you're deciding what to drink with your meals, choose water.

Because drinking too much water with a meal can affect your body's digestion, I suggest having a glass of water about ten to fifteen minutes before you eat. Then, during the meal, simply take small sips of water to help move the food from your mouth to your stomach. About fifteen minutes or so after the meal, you may have a little more water.

Buy Organic Whenever Possible and Wash Produce Thoroughly

Unless you have access to a local farm stand and know how your vegetables and fruits were grown, try to buy organic produce whenever possible. Although America has one of the safest food supplies in the world, we simply don't know how our foods were sprayed, grown, and handled from farm to table. Give yourself the best chance of eating the healthiest and most nutritious fresh foods possible by buying organic, and always wash your fruits and vegetables before eating.

Never Deprive Yourself

If you eat healthfully most of the time, you can indulge some of the time. One of the biggest mistakes people make that causes them to fail at dieting or eating healthier is doing too much too quickly, going to extremes, and denying themselves the foods they crave.

I'm not saying to eat whatever you want, whenever you want, in the amounts you want all the time. But if you are being fairly disciplined and watching what you eat during the week, and most of your meals are nutritious and healthy, then by all means allow yourself to have a little of your favorite indulgent or junk foods. I do!

HOW I SEE IT   I know firsthand what it feels like to deprive yourself. I also know just how much it can backfire. We boxers go to great lengths to make weight. Not only do we diet down during the weeks before a weigh in, we also dehydrate ourselves. As soon as I step off the scale after a weigh-in, I find myself guzzling water and pigging out on all of the foods I've been trying so hard not to eat! I need to make weight because my career is on the line.

You do not need to diet down to an unreasonably slender weight for your career. For your personal sanity and your weight-loss success, I recommend that you never aim for an artificial number on the scale. Don't starve yourself to reach that number. Rather than using the scale to judge your success, use your habits. Change your eating habits gradually over time, allowing your body to slowly find its natural and healthy weight.

Don't Think of It as Dieting; You Are Changing Your Eating Habits

You'd be surprised at how just replacing a word can change your life. Take the word *diet*. I don't know about you, but whenever I hear that word, I feel as if I'm forcing myself to do something I don't like, something that'll be hard work. In the past, diets have brought me more failure and unhappiness than success and joy. A diet just doesn't sound like very much fun. Don't you agree?

Good! Now we're on the same page. So, let's get rid of the *diet* word and replace it with something that sounds and feels better. Perhaps "eating well"? I like the words "eating well" because they mean two things: when I'm eating well, I'm eating nutritiously, and when I'm eating well, I'm enjoying the foods I eat.

Go ahead and choose your own word or words if you like. Just make them fun and inviting whenever you say or think about them.

Learn to Read Food Labels

Develop the confidence you need to decide whether to buy a product or to leave it on the shelf. Forget about what the fancy-looking label on the front of the package says or looks like. Always pay more attention to the back of the package.

For years, advertisers and food manufacturers have bombarded us with catchphrases like "lower fat," "reduced sodium," "⅓ less calories," and so on. On the front of the package, that sounds great. Yet when you turn the package around, you see that "lower fat" is only a gram or two of fat less (but it can still contain huge amounts of fat!), "reduced sodium" still means more sodium than you would need for two meals, or "⅓ less calories" is only ⅓ less than the regular version of the food, which is loaded with excess calories and which makes ⅓ less still excessive. And the list goes on.

Be smart about what you put into your body. You have only so much time to exercise and work off extra calories. Give yourself a huge head start by not overeating in the first place.

6

Mental Toughness, in and out of the Ring

As I mentioned earlier in this book, knowing what to eat and how to exercise are only part of the formula for achieving better health and a leaner, sexier body. In addition to knowing *what* to do, you also must find the resolve to *do* it. That's what this chapter will teach you.

I learned at a young age how important discipline was to attaining my goals. It's been a lesson I've never forgotten. So often in life, the difference between someone who achieves success and another who doesn't is that the person with discipline will take action to create a result. Others merely think or talk about their dreams but don't act to make them come true.

As a boxer, many times I didn't want to do all of the road-running work, sparring, bag work, rope work, weight workouts, and conditioning that I knew I needed to do to reach a level of conditioning that would enable me to win. But my discipline always propelled me to do whatever was necessary. I chose not to listen to that lazy voice inside my head and instead to obey the champion's voice. That's how I not only met my previous levels of conditioning and skills, but went beyond them. I want you to think this way, too. Start to see yourself as a champion, a world champion, who can create any result or have any experience you want, and who easily has the discipline to follow your inner voice telling you what to do and how.

Here's a lesson about discipline that will make it even easier for you to grasp. The more disciplined you are, the more rewards you will experience in every area of your life. In fact, performing only one disciplined act will bring you multiple rewards. To accomplish anything in life, you must first take action, because if you never start, it's absolutely certain you won't arrive. And if action is the prerequisite to all success, then discipline is the engine that puts action into gear.

The more disciplined you are, the more you will accomplish and the faster you will accomplish it. Yet being disciplined not only helps you accomplish your goal, it also brings you many other rewards simply from performing that one disciplined act.

For example, let's consider the discipline of eating well. Perhaps you want to lose 10 pounds of fat, so you make one disciplined change in your life: you begin to eat more nutritious foods. Look at what happens as a result of that one disciplined act:

1. Your body now has more energy because of the healthy foods you are eating.
2. You feel better and not so sluggish.
3. Your digestion has improved.
4. You sleep better.
5. Your complexion is better.
6. You're saving money because, on average, it costs you less to eat healthy foods than processed and junk foods.
7. You're getting leaner each week—losing the fat and keeping your lean muscle tissue—because your diet now contains the proper ratio of protein, carbohydrates, and fat.

8. Because you feel and look better, this raises your self-confidence and enhances your self-image and self-esteem. You also grow more comfortable being naked in front of your partner, and this can lead to a better sex life.

9. All of this enriches your relationships with others, you become more patient with your kids, your job performance improves, you begin to believe that you can set goals and achieve them.

10. Because you see and feel the results that follow just *one* disciplined act, eating more nutritiously, you now have a strong desire to begin an exercise program, which will change your body and the way you feel even quicker—not to mention bring more rewards.

Take a good look at that list: ten benefits and rewards just by performing one disciplined act! You can experience the same number of rewards—and, no doubt, a lot more—by being disciplined in every area of your life.

There seems to be a unwritten creed that says, "The harder you are on yourself (the more disciplined you are), the easier life will be. Whereas the easier you are on yourself (the less disciplined you are), the harder life will be."

The choice has always been yours. Choose discipline, and get ready for all of the rewards that follow.

Mental Strategies for Calm and Power

Let me give you some suggestions on how to strengthen your inner power and minimize the outside influences that can erode this power. Although you don't need to practice all of these mental habits, I recommend that you at least try them and experiment with whatever works best for you.

I first began using the strategies in this chapter to help myself stay calm and focused in the ring. Eventually, I also applied these techniques to other aspects of my life. For one, dealing with my kids; some days, it seems unbearable, and I don't know how I stay sane!

These tips even help me stay calm in rush-hour traffic, which is so common here in California. Rather than getting into altercations with the other drivers, I've learned to remain peaceful and focused, and my drive goes more smoothly as a result.

Meditation

A couple of times a day, I sit in a quiet spot, close my eyes, and imagine myself in a happy place. For me, the happy place is usually the beach. (Yours might be somewhere else.) I try to imagine every detail, from the smell of the salt air to the warmth of the sun against my skin and the sounds of the waves breaking on the shore line. I even imagine the sensation of sand on my feet. This helps me to focus and quickly create an inner sense of contentment so that I can shed the frustration and stress that tend to prevent my getting anything accomplished. I meditate before every fight.

Deep Breathing

The best boxers are able to stay calm and collected in the ring, constantly analyzing their opponents for weaknesses and mentally strategizing their every move. When I first began my career, maintaining this mind-set was a challenge. Whenever I walked to the ring, my heart began to race. To help myself stay calm, I started to practice deep breathing. I do these exercises several times a day. I simply take a break from whatever I'm doing and sit down and breathe. Then, whenever I feel myself tense up (such as when battling other drivers on a freeway), or when my kids make me want to scream, I quickly turn to my breath to calm myself down, and it works terrifically.

DID YOU KNOW THAT... It's a great idea after a workout to drink diluted fruit juice. Try mixing half a can of seltzer or carbonated water with half a can of fruit juice. Not only will you reduce your calories by 50 percent, but it will help your body better absorb the carbohydrates in the juice, to replenish the muscle fuel (glycogen) your body used during the workout. It also tastes delicious.

Alternate Nostril Breathing

Sit comfortably in a quiet place where you won't be disturbed. Take a couple of deep breaths. Use your thumb to close off your right nostril, inhaling deeply and slowly through your left nostril. Then open your right nostril and use your middle finger to close the left. Exhale slowly and fully out the right side. Inhale through the right, exhale out the left, and then repeat.

1. Inhale left.
2. Exhale right.
3. Inhale right.
4. Exhale left.
5. Repeat.

Breath Retention

Sit comfortably in a quiet place where you won't be disturbed. Take a couple of deep breaths. Then fully inhale, feeling your tummy expand forward, your rib cage outward, and your chest upward. When you can inhale no more air, hold your breath for a count of 4. Then fully exhale. When you can exhale no further, hold for a count of 4. Repeat this a few times. As you practice, increase the length of time you hold the inhalation and the exhalation.

Mental Power Boosters

Focus on self-control, not on controlling other people. The one thing you do have complete control over is your thoughts. Regardless of how hard other people may try, they can never control or take away your power to think, choose, and be, unless you give them permission to do so.

The greatest philosophers and thinkers throughout the ages have always said that to know ourselves is one of the greatest aspirations we can have, and to control ourselves (and direct our lives to whatever paths we choose) is one of the most important things we will ever do in life.

What does that mean for you right here, right now, today? Plenty. It means that from this day forward, you will let go of the need and desire to control what others think, say, or do and simply let them be. It means that you will now use all of that extra power you had previously directed toward being overly concerned about others and will channel that power into thinking, dreaming, and becoming what you most desire, regardless of what others say, think, or do.

My mantra for releasing my urge to control other people and outside situations is the Serenity Prayer. I'm amazed at how effective it is in helping me refocus and change my emotions and outlook.

Remember what I told you earlier about the amazing power and rewards you'll receive from being disciplined? Well, my friend, just what do you think self-control is? It's simply another form of discipline. And what happens when you take one disciplined action? You reap countless rewards. The same thing will happen when you add more self-control in your life.

Think Like a Boxer, in and out of the Ring

A fundamental lesson I learned was not to confront anyone when I am mad. I wait a day or two, so that I don't say something out of anger that I may not intend. Later, when I feel calm enough, I confront the person and explain how I feel. The same principle applies in a boxing match: when you get angry, you lose control.

I try not to use words like "you made me feel" because no one makes you feel anything. You allow yourself to feel like that. You let that person affect you. Don't be a victim! If you can point to at least five people who are jerks, chances are you might be the one with the problem! Don't think that everyone is against you and is talking about you. This happens a lot in the workplace, no matter what your job is, even in boxing. Also, don't let other people's bad moods determine your mood.

I used to wake up in the morning and gauge my kids' or husband's mood, and I'd allow this to influence my own mood. If they were happy, so was I. If they were cranky, then I was, too. It was crazy. I had to learn how to separate myself from them and not be codependent. This is extremely difficult to do when it's with someone you love.

You have to learn how to let go. Again, the Serenity Prayer has worked wonders in my life, and it could for you, too.

Take Control of Power-Eroding Life Circumstances

Life happens each and every day, and not a single day will be exactly the same as the one before it. Things change. People change. Friends change. Families change. Jobs and careers change. Your pattern of eating changes. Your exercise changes. *Everything* in this life is always in a state of constant change. And when you get right down to it, the only thing that doesn't change is change!

So, what will you do about all of the changes in your life? Have fun with them! First, you will no longer get so freaked out when change occurs. The reason many people are scared and uncomfortable when confronted by change is that they feel that they're losing control—that is, self-control.

Some people grew up in families where they always had to be in control of everything. They carried those beliefs into their adult lives. They were taught that before they made any decision or took any action, they had to know in advance all of the steps they would take and the events that would happen as a result. But life doesn't work like that.

Four years ago, could you have told me in advance everything that would happen in your life that would enable you to get to where and who you are today? Of course, you couldn't have. And neither could I or anyone else. In the same vein, don't you see how silly it is to waste time thinking about all of the workouts you will do, the meals you will eat, the actions you will take, the experiences you will have, and the lessons you will learn until you reach where you want to go?

Take things one day at a time. Live by the conviction that just for *today* you will eat well. You don't know about tomorrow, but *today* you will eat nutritious foods. Take it one day at a time for the rest of your life. Just for today you will accomplish this or that and will do it well.

Take the pressure off yourself. Throw off the weight you've been lugging around all of these years by needing to know what will happen, how it will happen, and when, because that prevents you from following your dreams and achieving your goals.

Dream the dream. Plan the goal. Listen to your inner voice, which gives you inspiration and ideas so that you can make plans and take action. All that you need to do is move to the next step, and you will know what that step is by trusting yourself.

Find Your Inner Passion

I firmly believe that we are all born with gifts, talents, and abilities that allow us to follow our dreams and become successful at them. If you want to look and feel better, then you absolutely can, no doubt about it. You've got a body, just like anyone else who's in great shape, and all that you need to do is take the right action (such as eating better and exercising effectively), and you will reach your goal. That's the way I and many others have done it.

Stop for moment and think about what in your life brings you the greatest joy and happiness. Besides your family, what is it that you do (or perhaps haven't done in a long time) that makes you feel good whenever you do it? Whatever it is (there are no limits, and nothing is too outrageous or silly!), take that thought a little further and imagine what it would be like if your life was filled with doing what you love. How would that make you feel? Pretty great, huh?

Do you see where I'm going with this? I'm taking you out of your rut, your comfort zone, and we're dusting the cobwebs off your dreams and bringing them out into the open for you to see and get excited about.

One of the biggest killers of your dreams is imagining how other people would respond if you revealed your deepest desires. A false need for others' approval and validation of your dream will destroy your happiness simply because you believe that someone else's opinion of your life is more important than your own. Does that make any sense to you? Of course, it doesn't. So let go of the need to get other people's approval before you begin living your dream.

This is *your* precious life. It has been given only to you. It's your gift.

Follow your passion. Follow your bliss. Follow your dream, and your life will never be the same.

Take the Risks That Will Change Your Life for the Better

Each time I stepped into the ring as a boxer, I encountered huge risks. I could have gotten injured. I could have lost the bout (and I have in the past, but I learned how to accept it, learned from my mistakes, and moved on). So many things could have happened that weren't under my control. But that's okay. I decided to take those risks and to focus on the rewards. I became a world champion by doing so, and I believe you can, too—a champion at whatever you love to do.

Fighting is my passion, and the money didn't matter because I was doing what I loved. It's great that I am paid well for it, but money has never made me a happy person. I believe that if you do what you love and your basic needs are met, nothing else matters.

DID YOU KNOW THAT... For better digestion, eat a piece of papaya before your meals. Papaya contains an enzyme called *papain* that helps break down the proteins in the foods you eat and helps your body better use the nutrients you give it. For many people, a slice of tomato or pineapple works well, too.

Listen to your heart and follow wherever its passion and desire lead you. Keep your eyes focused only on the goal, and move your thoughts, actions, and life in only one direction: forward to your goal and dream.

Forget your past, what's behind you. Don't get distracted by what's to your left or your right. All that matters is the here and now. You need to make the present moment count so that tomorrow you will be where you want to be. This very moment and every moment should count because all we have is today.

We never know what tomorrow will bring. Once I began to concentrate on today, the here and now, I was able to appreciate what was in front of me, instead of thinking "Tomorrow I'll do this" or "I can't wait 'til this happens." I used to wish my fights would come and go quickly because I was so nervous that I wanted to get them over with. But then when each fight was finished, I felt sad that it was over.

So I stopped wishing my fights and the rest of my life away. I began to live in the moment, knowing that this instant in time would never exist again: the crowd cheering, the excitement of the fight. One day I would be old, and this would be all over. So I decided to enjoy every moment, even my nervousness.

I love this saying: "If you have one foot in the past and one in the future, you're pissing on the present." In life, you will find that risk and reward are equal. Little risk equals little, if any, reward. The bigger the risk, the bigger the reward.

Goal Achieving by the New You— See Yourself As You Want to Be

The more you believe in yourself, the more success you will experience. I'll bet that if I could attach a "belief gauge" to you, a gadget that would measure the amount of belief you have in yourself, on a scale from 1 to 100, I could tell just by looking at that number what kind of life you've lived so far and how much success and what kinds of experiences you've had.

Years ago, if someone had put such a gauge on me, it would've shown a lack of belief; lots of frustration, doubt, and uncertainty; and few rewards and little success. Then things started to change. Not all at once, mind you, but slowly, I began to notice a shift in how I looked at my life and felt about myself. Slowly and steadily, I began to dream bigger dreams, set larger goals, and envision myself as someone greater than who I was.

I've always dreamed big; I just had some roadblocks I had to get around first. When I was twelve, I dreamed I was Rocky! My father once told me that if I pretended to be someone long enough, I would become that person. So I started to pretend that I had great self-esteem because even though I may not have felt it at the time, I thought that if I pretended long enough, maybe one day I would.

This was the 1970s, when the models were extremely thin, and I weighed 80 pounds, so kids said I was fat. Okay, this was in the third grade, and maybe I was a little pudgy. I was very shy, and the kids picked on me a lot. As a result, I spent most of my time daydreaming.

My mother, born and raised in Mexico, was very spiritual because of her Indian background. She always told me to be careful of my thoughts because they would become reality. I really believed it, and I actually imagined myself opening for Oscar de la Hoya. I told people I would do it even before it happened!

I told everyone I would sign with Don King before it happened. I told people I was going to build a house, and then I did. I announced that I was going to be on the cover of *Playboy* before the magazine asked me to, and I proved that Latinas were just as hot as any American woman. I did everything I said I would do because I believed it and put the plan in motion.

I started to think of who I *wanted* to be. As the image of my new self grew stronger and more powerful, a new understanding of life arose in my mind. My life began to open up. I saw and envisioned things as they could be and not as they were. New possibilities and ideas popped into my brain, erasing the old limitations about how much money and what type of experiences I could have. In their place sprang up dreams with no limits. No walls. No fences. As fully as I could imagine something, I could become it.

In a short time, I was amazed at how much every part of my life changed for the better. The sky and my imagination were now my only limits. I loved it, and I still do to this day! It can be the same for you.

Becoming a new you does not mean having a fake self or living a false life. Instead, you are finally allowing your amazing essence, which has always been inside of you, to come out and play, dream dreams, achieve goals, have the experiences you desire, and live your life to the fullest and on your own terms, without ever needing again to ask anyone's permission whether it's okay.

Give yourself that gift. Allow the greater you to come out. The new vistas, destinations, and experiences you're about to enjoy will bring such happiness and love to your life.

THE
EXTRA EDGE

7

Optional Supplements

Over the years, many people have asked me about nutritional supplements: which to take, which to avoid, the latest incredible pill or powder, and so on. Open any page of a fitness, health, or body-building magazine and you'll see ad after ad for supplements, as if they were the answers to your nutritional prayers.

Many people swear by supplements, and some of them do have a place in your food pantry, but most do not. Here's why. You need to understand that supplements are, as the word says, *a supplement to something*—as in, a good nutritious eating plan. Supplements will not make up for poor eating habits, no matter how many you take.

Your body needs nutrients from a variety of foods, such as grains, meats, dairy products, vegetables, and fruits. Your body has evolved to use these foods as its fuel and source of nutrients. Yet somewhere along the way, our lives grew too busy, and the messages from many supplement makers became blurred.

Over the years, I've known and worked with top-level athletes and have spoken to many scientists and researchers. Most of them say:

- Supplements may work for some people but not nearly as well for others.

- For people whom supplements benefit, many report only *minimal* improvements in their performance.

- And for individuals who swear by supplements, an even smaller number of them may notice a change in performance, but that change usually lasts only a short time and can be quite expensive to maintain.

- When you look at the cost-to-performance/results ratio, supplements are expensive.

- Many people say they have to take supplements often and in high dosages—quite often higher than the doses listed in the magazines—in order to get any noticeable results.

- Your money is more wisely spent if you buy good, healthy foods.

I've learned that a few key supplements can give you the energy you need to improve your fitness. They also can bolster your health and, I've personally found, help prevent colds and the flu. Like anything, however, be it exercise or eating, too much can be counterproductive and even harmful. So, when you're deciding which supplements to take and how much, it's always a good idea to talk to your doctor.

That said, however, I'd like you to consider taking the following essential supplements as part of your overall nutrition program.

Multivitamin/Mineral Supplement

As much as we like to think we're getting all of the vitamins and minerals we need each day, in the right amounts and ratios, simply from the foods we eat, the truth is that many people are not. On some days, we may find it easy to eat five servings of vegetables, and on other days we're lucky if we eat one. Often, we're so busy with work, kids, school, and other activities that we don't have time to prepare completely nutritious meals, so we head to the nearest drive-thru restaurant and pick up something for the road.

That's why I've always taken a good vitamin and mineral supplement, and I recommend this to others. It doesn't have to cost a fortune or contain exotic ingredients and extracts that sound too good to be true. It simply needs to give your body all of the basics. Think of vitamins and minerals as the metabolic spark plugs that help your body's engine to fire and run optimally and to use the foods you give it more effectively for everything from energy to digestion, repair, and recuperation.

People who take multivitamin/mineral supplements all have their favorite brands. and I'm not paid to endorse any of them. I can, however, recommend Costco's vitamin/mineral supplement. It is excellent and offers quite a bang for your buck. I suggest that you simply find one you like and take it each day.

Some people ask me how they should take a multivitamin/mineral supplement. I take mine only once a day, in the morning, right in the middle of breakfast. If you've ever taken vitamins and minerals on an empty stomach, then you know the taste is just plain horrible. It stays with you as a metallic aftertaste for the rest of the day.

Always take your supplements with food. I've found that my body makes better use of the nutrients that way, and it leaves no unpleasant aftertaste. Take only one multivitamin/mineral supplement per day. That's all you need.

Powdered Vitamin C

You can find vitamin C in various forms, from pills to liquids, chewables, and powder. At the end of the day, it's all vitamin C. The difference is which type you prefer to take and how it affects your body. I've tried them all and found that powdered vitamin C gets into my bloodstream quicker than pills and chewables do. I can also add powdered C to the foods I eat or the meals I prepare, to amp up their nutritional punch.

With nutrition, one size doesn't fit all, but here's a tip that seems to work well for a lot of people. Many have found that simply adjusting the time of day that they eat carbohydrates greatly affects their weight. The key is to eat most of your high-carbohydrate foods early in the day (for example, from the morning through 1 or 2 p.m.), then taper them down, and from early afternoon through the evening, do just the opposite and make most of the foods you eat protein. Some people say that their bodies more effectively use the carbs for energy early in the day, as compared to eating them later in the day or at night. Remember this carbohydrate formula: eat the most carbs in the morning, less in the afternoon, and the least at night. Experiment to see how this works for you.

When I'm training hard, my body needs more nutrients for energy, recuperation, and recovery. Many times during the year, I might train more than four hours a day, when all of my boxing, gym exercises, and other training are combined. Simply taking the recommended daily amount of nutrients and eating the suggested number of calories for my age and body weight will not cut it. My body needs more, and believe me, when you're training effectively and intensely, you *can* feel the difference.

Add some extra vitamin C to your diet. Try all four types to see how they affect your body. Everyone's body reacts differently to various forms of the same nutrients.

Calcium

A lot of women don't get enough calcium. Some like dairy products and have no problem tolerating lactose, and for them, dairy (low-fat/nonfat, please) can be a good way to get the daily recommended amount of calcium (1,200 milligrams) for adults.

Others may not enjoy dairy products, might have milk allergies, cannot tolerate lactose, or may not enjoy the lactose-free versions. Although many foods contain calcium, unless you eat nutritionally balanced meals every day, you may not be getting the calcium your body needs.

The good news is that many nondairy foods also contain calcium. Here's a list of some of them:

- Peas
- Sardines
- Baked beans
- Sesame seeds
- Salmon
- Okra
- Almonds
- Collard greens

- Broccoli
- Tofu
- Bok choy
- Rhubarb
- Brussels sprouts
- Turnip greens
- White beans
- Spinach

If you're not able to get the recommended daily allowance of 1,200 mg of calcium each and every day, do yourself and your body a big favor and get a complete calcium supplement. (*Note:* Read the labels. Some of them advertise themselves as calcium supplements but don't give you the daily recommended amount.)

Glutamine

Let me tell you a little about this supplement. I started taking glutamine in 1994 when I was trying to gain weight to move into a different class for boxing. To gain weight, I had to build muscle, and this required a lot of weight lifting.

For athletes like me, who train two or more hours a day, such tough sessions can reduce immunity and lead to a condition called "overtraining." I had heard from a number of pros that glutamine could bolster immunity and prevent overtraining syndrome, so I decided to try it. Amazingly, I haven't had a cold since! That's pretty incredible, given the fact that I have two children who attend school (schools are notorious germ factories) and who test my immunity every day.

For many years, scientists and researchers considered glutamine a nonessential amino acid, meaning that you could consume a diet that contained none of this protein building block and still remain healthy. A number of studies completed during the last ten years, however, have led many scientists to treat this amino acid with more respect.

Several studies show that this supplement helps very ill people (that is, people with heart disease, patients recovering from surgery, elderly people with breathing difficulties, children with muscular dystrophy, and so on) in a number of important ways. In children undergoing chemotherapy, the supplement reduced the need for antibiotics. In children with muscular dystrophy, glutamine supplementation preserved muscle mass. Interestingly, one study even found that supplementing with glutamine increased postmeal energy expenditure by 49 percent (or about 50 additional calories).

Glutamine supplementation appears to improve immunity and bolster muscle mass through its anti-inflammatory action. It reduces key markers of inflammation throughout the body, which allows the immune system to operate more effectively. It also improves digestion and directly enhances immune cell function. Not everyone needs glutamine, though.

I work out hard, exercising two or more hours a day. I also travel frequently, which puts my body through the stress of adapting to many different time zones. On top of that, I'm the mom of two teens. Need I say more? This type of lifestyle could easily leave me feeling drained and used up. When I take glutamine, however, I notice a difference in how energetic I feel.

You may benefit more from this supplement if any of the following are true:

- You frequently get too little sleep.
- You work the swing shift.
- You enjoy endurance exercise (working out for an hour or longer on most days).
- You underwent any type of surgery in the last year.
- You had a baby in the last two years (consult your pediatrician if you are breast-feeding).
- You suffer from frequent colds and flu.
- You feel tired, even when you wake up in the morning.

If any of these statements describe you, then you might want to give glutamine a try and see how it affects your body and feeling of well-being. It's certainly made a difference in my life.

8

Taking Fitness to the Next Level

To build a beautiful body and improve your health, you need not run marathons or spend hours in the gym. You only have to carry out the short and effective routines that I'm telling you about in this book.

That said, you may find that as you enhance your fitness and enrich your overall life, you'll want to take things to the next level. You may discover, as I have, that exercise becomes something you enjoy—something you *want* to do, rather than something you feel you *have* to do.

My fitness routine is an incredible stress reliever for me. It helps me calm down and keep everything in perspective. I actually feel as if I could not function without it. Working out makes my entire day go more smoothly.

It has also provided me with an incredible sense of self-confidence and empowerment. Boxing workouts in particular help to bring this out. Hitting the bag enables me to get my aggression out of my system. When I walk into the ring for a fight, I feel such a sense of empowerment and control.

So, if you begin to realize that you crave more, this chapter details some great ways to improve your fitness.

Always Do Something Different

I see this time and time again: people doing the same workouts, with the same exercises, the same weights, the same number of reps, on the same days and getting the same results—nothing!

If you're like me, you get bored really quickly by doing the same thing over and over and over. And when it comes to workouts and exercising, that kind of dull and boring routine can very quickly destroy your motivation and desire to exercise.

This is one reason I always do something a little different each time I work out. Sometimes these changes are radical and other times only slight adjustments and variations, but, most important, I have a different routine each and every time I work out, and so should you.

Once you start doing this, you'll feel more motivated. You'll actually look forward to your workouts, and the changes (even if they're slight) in exercises, rest periods, sets, number of reps, weights, and all of the other variables will keep your body responding, so that you get great results.

One training method I use throughout the year is called "periodization." It means using various workout structures (each one with its own rules for reps, weights, rest, etc.) during the twelve months of the year.

It's really simple. The legendary fitness icon Joe Weider, the founder and publisher of such magazines as *Shape* and *Muscle & Fitness*, put these structures into an easy-to-use and -understand format. He called his type of periodization "Cycle Training" and divided it into three distinct parts, which are described in the following sections.

Cycle Training

Many people who work out and train heavily all the time are at greater risk of injuring themselves than are those who cycle their training. The body is not a machine and can't be continually pushed and pounded without periods of rest and cycled training. Therefore, you should follow three distinct and separate cycles during the course of a year. They are:

- *The mass cycle*—Use moderate to heavy weights, give yourself no more than 90 seconds of rest between sets, and do 6 to 10 reps for the upper body and 8 to 20 reps for the lower body.

- *The power cycle*—Use heavy weights and do 3 to 8 reps for lower- and upper-body movements, with up to 3 minutes of rest between sets.

- *The cuts cycle*—Use light to moderate weights, do 12 to 25 reps, and take no more than 45 seconds of rest between sets.

To get the most from this type of training, stay on each cycle for 6 to 8 weeks, and then take 1 full week off from training before you move to the next cycle.

You may find yourself and your body in a rut, when it doesn't respond the way you'd like. I've learned that cycling my training (even

DID YOU KNOW THAT... Many people—especially women—are deficient in iron. They feel tired and run-down and wonder why. Lack of iron can be a major reason. Molasses is one of the best sources of iron and also contains other B vitamins. Molasses is made from the residue that is left when sugar is removed from sugar cane. Just a little molasses can do wonders for your energy and health. Find the darkest molasses available at the store, and add a bit to muffins, waffles, and whole-grain breads. One tablespoon of molasses (depending on the kind) can provide up to 75 percent of your daily iron allowance.

if only briefly, when I can't commit to a full 6- to 8-week cycle) does wonders to take my body to the next level of fitness.

A Great Way to Work Out Year Round

When I'm training for a fight, I usually do cardio and weights during the day and my boxing training at night. Cardio consists of running either hills or the stairs. I use light to moderate weights and break the exercises down into which body parts I focus on: chest, shoulders, and triceps on one day; back and biceps the next day; and then legs the third day. I do abs four times a week. (For more on how to figure out the right size of weights for you, see the list in the section titled "My Favorite Weight-Training Exercises" later in this chapter.)

I work out for three days straight, then take a day off, then three days, one day off, and so on. I get one day off a week. At night, I warm up with the jump rope, then hit the mitts, go over drills or strategy, or spar. When I'm not in training for a fight, I don't do the boxing training at night. For exercises, I like to do 4 sets per exercise, with 10 to 12 reps in each set. For abs, I'll do a total of 200 reps.

A normal person does not have to work out with weights three times a week. You can substitute one of your cardio/weight training days for boxing. It's a great way to get your cardio and muscle toning in at the same time.

Level Two Workout with the Knockout

If you've completed my Level One Knockout Workout Plan in chapter 4 and want to take your fitness to the next level, here are some of my favorite workouts for the advanced exerciser.

This first workout incorporates elements of boxing, weight training, martial arts, stretching, and mental calming. I'd like you to perform 3 or 4 sets of each exercise, with at least 10 reps per set.

First, the warm-up.

The Warm-Up

I recommend jumping rope to warm up and get the blood flowing. Jump ropes are easy to find at a gym, and they're small enough and cheap enough to have one in your own home.

Begin with 2 to 3 sets of 25 reps. As your conditioning improves, then go for 50 to 100 reps per set. Rest no longer than a minute between sets. Since this is a warm-up, be sure not to do too much jump rope or do it so intensely that it affects your main workout.

For the Legs and the Glutes

Mia's Move for the Front Legs: The Squat

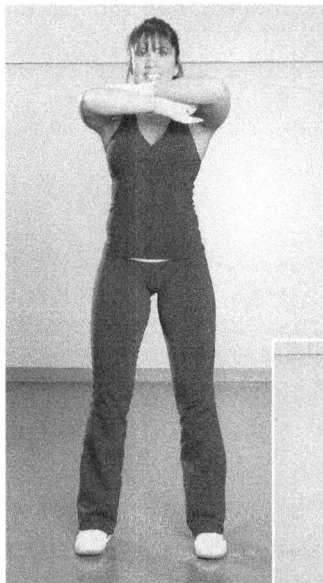

THE MOVE

One of the best exercises you can do for your legs is the squat. This exercise not only targets the front leg muscles (the quads), but works the hamstrings, the glutes, and the lower back at the same time. Proper form is essential when performing the squat. You want your upper body to be upright, with your head up as you look forward, and the upper part of your legs to be roughly parallel to the floor when you reach the bottom of the movement. Be sure to keep your knees in line with your toes, and don't let your knees go forward over your toes at the lowest position.

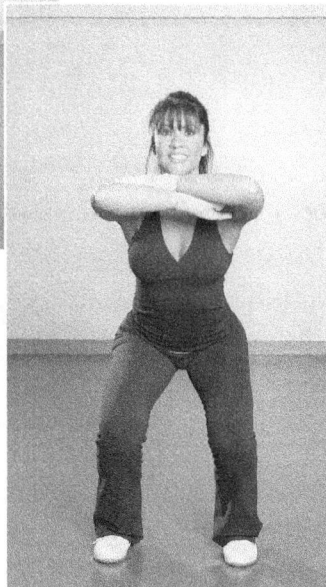

HOW TO DO IT

Stand erect with your head up as you look forward, and place your feet about shoulder width apart and toes pointing straight in front of you. Keep your abdominals pulled in. Extend your arms out in front of your body, with your elbows bent. Cross your hands so they are resting on opposite

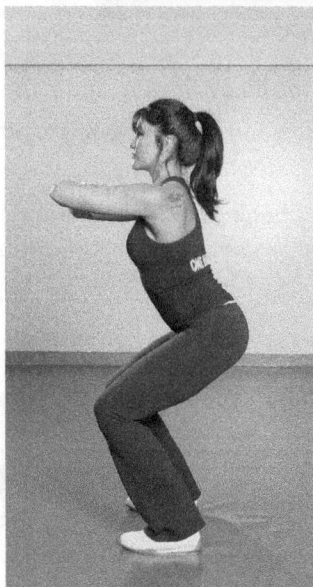

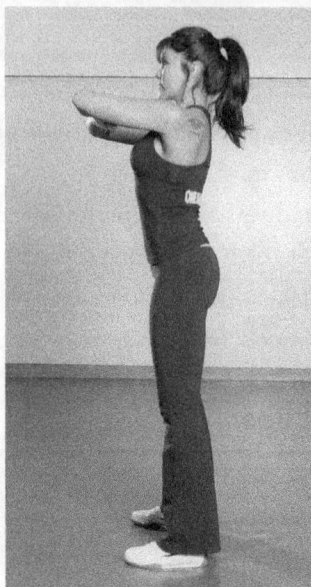

elbows. While keeping your arms in this position, shift your weight back onto your heels, inhale with a deep breath, and bend your knees as you squat down. Pretend there's a chair behind you and you're about to sit in it as you lower yourself into a squatting position. Go no lower than having your thighs parallel to the floor. Stopping a little higher than parallel is just fine. As you get ready to return to the top starting position, exhale while squeezing your glutes as you bring your body up. Go for 2 to 3 sets of 12 to 15 reps.

Quick tip: Keep your chest raised from start to finish, and don't sit lower than the upper-legs-parallel-to-floor point or let your knees move forward past your toes.

Mia's Move for the Legs and the Glutes: The Walking Lunge

THE MOVE

The walking lunge is one of my favorite exercises to target not only the fronts and back of the legs, but also the glutes. I see many women doing lunges, but very few do them correctly. Or perhaps I should say "effectively." As with any exercise, it's easy to just go through the motions, but that's not what you want to do. You want results, and you'll get them by focusing directly on the muscles and using great form. The good news is, you don't even need to use weights (your body weight alone is enough!) to get terrific results.

HOW TO DO IT

Begin by standing with your legs and feet together. Keep your chest up, your upper body erect, your back straight, and your abdominals pulled in, as you look straight ahead. With your left foot, take a big step forward. Now drop your right

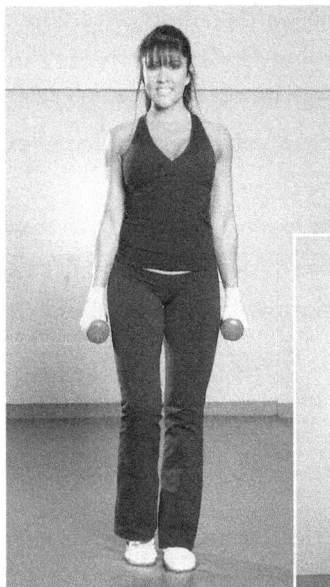

knee down toward the ground and try to keep it directly under your body and as closely in a direct line with your upper body as you can. Be sure to keep your upper body upright, with your arms straight down at your sides, and to look forward while you are in the lowered position.

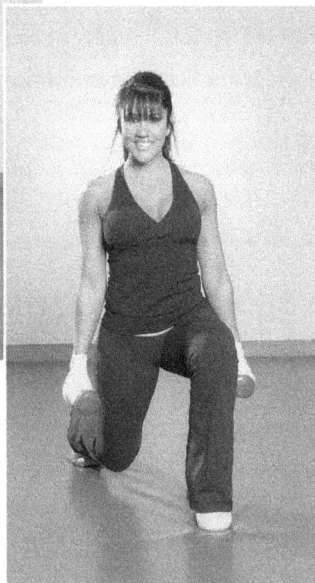

Now bring your upper body to a standing position and move your right leg forward, with your left leg down and directly under your body and the left knee almost touching the floor as you repeat the same sequence with the opposite leg.

Keep moving forward (one leg, then the other) until you reach the end of the room or someplace where you can turn around, and repeat everything for your next set. You will inhale as you lower your back leg and exhale as you come up. Go for 2 to 3 sets of 15 to 20 reps each.

Mia's Move for the Glutes and the Hamstrings: The Leg Raise

THE MOVE

Leg raises require no special equipment and no weights. They can be done anywhere. They really make the glutes and hamstrings burn, and if you want tight glutes and great-looking muscles in the back of your legs, that's a good thing. This is a really simple move, so let's get started!

HOW TO DO IT

Begin on the floor on your hands and knees. Keep your back straight and your neck in line with your spine. Keep your abs tight. Start the move by bending your knee and lifting your right leg up behind you as you straighten the leg and knee. Raise the leg up to a level that's comfortable, but also to a point where you really feel the exercise targeting the glutes and the backs of the legs.

At the top of the move, hold your leg in the upward contracted position for one count before returning to the starting position. Do 2 to 3 sets of 12 to 15 reps before you switch to the other side. Inhale before you begin the move, then exhale as you raise your leg up, and inhale again as you bring your leg back to the starting position.

Just be patient and don't push yourself too far too fast by trying to raise your leg higher than is comfortable. You'll find that as you continue doing this exercise as part of your routine, your flexibility will improve, thereby increasing your range of motion.

For the Legs and Core

Mia's Move for the Glutes and the Hamstrings: The Roundhouse Kick

THE MOVE

Kicking and punching are such great moves for your body. You can do them just about anywhere. You don't need a gym membership, weights, or machines, and since kicks and punches use your body weight, you're limited only by your flexibility and endurance level. Not all of us started out with great flexibility and a wide range of motion. Like any physical activity, the roundhouse kick takes practice and a little time and effort to perfect, but progress will come quickly if you follow these tips.

HOW TO DO IT

Begin the move with your body in a standing position, your feet about shoulder width apart. Keep your body weight equally distributed so that you feel balanced and the center of gravity is directly underneath you. Keep your arms up in boxing stance, fists beside your cheeks, as you allow your upper body to flex and move to the opposite side of your raised kicking right leg, so that the side of your right knee is almost parallel to the floor.

Flex your right heel and bring it back toward your body and in close and in line with your hip. Now you're ready to execute the strike position. Extend your right leg outward as you snap your foot horizontally forward, toward your target, using the top of your foot as the strike point.

From the extended forward position, your right leg will now move around in a half-circular motion toward the rear of your body as you bend your knee while retracting your foot and then slowly lower the foot down until you're in a standing position.

Do 2 to 3 sets of 12 to 15 reps before switching to the other side. You will inhale before you begin the move, then exhale as you raise your leg up, and inhale as you bring your leg back to the starting position.

Quick tip: Remember to keep your knees bent and don't kick above hip height until you are really comfortable with the move. (See the photos in chapter 4, page 68.)

For the Upper Body

Mia's Move for the Chest and the Arms: The Push-Up

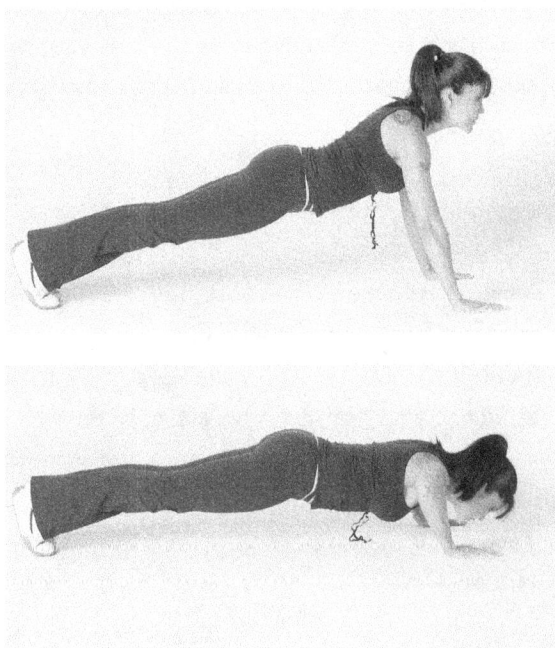

THE MOVE

You probably think of push-ups as a guy thing. Soldiers do them. We did them in PE class in school. But not many people do them as part of their workouts, and they're missing a great move that produces excellent results in a short period of time.

Of course, you may not be superstrong and in good enough shape to do push-ups with only your feet and hands touching the floor (that's why you can let your knees touch the floor until you get strong enough!), but I promise that if you can do just one push-up, it won't be long before you'll be able to do many more.

HOW TO DO IT

Begin the move by getting down on the floor on your hands and knees. Now raise your body off your knees and onto your toes and hands, as you stretch your legs straight out behind you. Make sure your hands remain positioned directly under your shoulders with your fingers pointing forward. Keep your abdominal muscles contracted and your spine in a straight neutral position.

As you slowly lower your body, inhale and bend your elbows. Your body should be a few inches above the floor and not resting on it. This position keeps your muscles contracted and working. Once you reach the bottom of the move, exhale as you push your body back up to the starting position. Go for 2 to 3 sets of 8 to 12 reps.

Quick tip: If you feel any pain or strain in your lower back or if your triceps aren't yet strong enough to do the full move, you can modify the push-up by bending your knees and performing the exercise on your knees and hands until you build strength.

Mia's Move for the Backs of the Arms: The Triceps Dip

THE MOVE

Here is another great exercise that's very effective and uses only your body weight. It's called the triceps dip, and it works the muscles in the backs of your arms, called the triceps.

Since you'll bend your elbows during the move, as you allow your body to come up and down, I highly recommend that you warm up the elbow area first before doing any triceps work.

A great elbow/triceps warm-up is to stand with your body facing a wall. Begin by standing roughly 1 to 2 feet away from the wall. Place your hands out on front of you on the wall at about shoulder-width. While keeping your body erect, allow your elbows to bend and your body to move closer to the wall. As your upper body reaches near the wall, contract your triceps and straighten your arms, locking out your elbows so that your upper body is in the starting position. Do 1 to 2 warm-up sets of 8 to 12 reps per set.

Now you're ready for the triceps dips.

HOW TO DO IT

To do the exercise, you'll need a bench or a straight-backed chair. Sit on the bench or the chair, and place your hands on the edge of the seat with your fingers facing forward. Keep your upper body erect, your abs tight, and look straight ahead. With a slight bend in your knees, extend your legs out in front of you and place your feet on the floor for stability.

Slowly bend your arms and lower your body in front of the bench or the chair so that your glutes/butt are below bench level. Don't let your shoulders scrunch

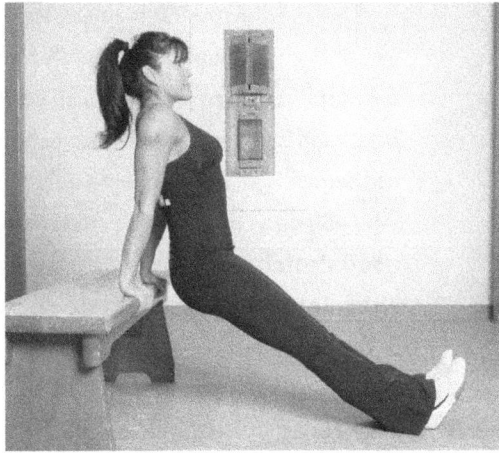
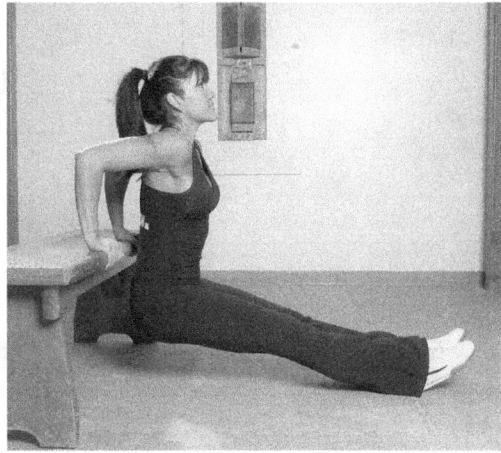

up to your ears or don't go so low that you place strain on your shoulders. Go down only as far as is comfortable, but you will really feel the exercise in the backs of your arms. Straighten your arms as you raise your body back up. Do 2 to 3 sets of 8 to 12 reps.

Quick tip: For safety and greater effectiveness, keep your elbows close to your body throughout the movement.

The Stretch

Mia's Move for Stretching the Upper Body, the Obliques, and the Legs: The Saddle Stretch

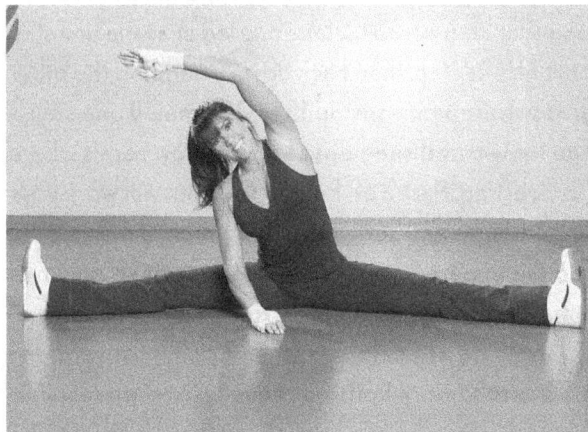

THE MOVE

Although many of us think of stretching as part of the cooldown, stretching can and should be done before the workout begins or after the main workout is completed. You can also do stretching between sets, with various body parts, and any time in the workout when you'd like more flexibility and increased blood flow to the body part that you're working.

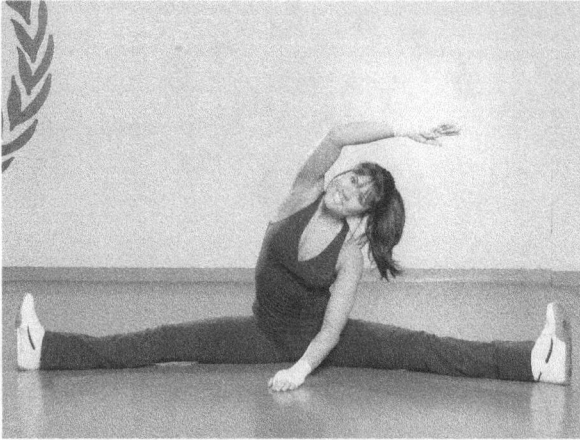

The saddle stretch is great for the upper body, the obliques, and the legs. All that it requires is that you sit on the floor and separate your legs as wide as they will go. Now, how easy is that? And you don't have to do a split to get a good stretch, either. Never force your body into anything that feels too extreme. Simply separate your legs to the point that's comfortable but where you feel a nice stretch.

HOW TO DO IT

Keep your abdominals pulled in and your back straight. With your right hand on the floor in front of you, stretch your left arm over your head. Now lean over and into the stretch by bending only from the waist. Make sure that your left upper arm remains next to your ear and that your upper body does not fall forward.

DID YOU KNOW THAT... Traveling and staying in a hotel no longer have to be bad for your body if you know some of the tricks to working out on the road. Here's a great one for your legs, butt, calves, and heart. Forget the elevator and find the stairs. Part 1 is the stride, which works the fronts and the backs of the legs and the butt. Just as you'd do lunges or step aerobics, take one leg at a time and step up to the next higher step, then back down. Then step the other leg up, then down. Repeat nonstop 15 to 20 times. If one step is easy, then go for two or three steps at a time. Now here's where things get interesting. Part 2 of the stair workout will work your inner and outer thighs and butt. Instead of going forward up the stairs as you did in part 1, you'll do it sideways. Take only one step at a time because in your ability to do lateral (sideways) motion, you won't be as flexible as when moving forward and backward. Be sure to work both legs equally for even results.

Hold the stretch for several counts, then repeat by bending to the other side and stretching your right arm, while having your left hand on the floor in front of you. Don't bounce! You can repeat the stretch several more times or bend forward from the hips and place your arms out in front of your body.

Quick tip: Always remember that a cooldown after an intense workout is beneficial for your body, as it helps your muscles relax and helps distribute the metabolic waste products (such as lactic acid) that build up in the body from your workout, moving them out and away from the muscles you worked. Stretching also provides these health benefits:

- It reduces the risk of injuries.
- It increases mobility, range of motion, and muscle suppleness and coordination.
- It improves nutrient, oxygen, and blood flow to the muscles and the tissues.
- It calms your mind and increases mental clarity.

My Favorite Ways to Exercise

I love running on hills (if you are a beginner, you can simply walk), running up stairs (beginners can walk), and jumping rope. As a marathon runner, I have sometimes run 15 miles a day. I also like to run up stairs really fast in 3-minute intervals, with a 1-minute rest in between. It's good for me because it mimics the pace of an actual fight.

I do cardio for my heart and for the conditioning it gives my body; I don't do it to lose weight. Although cardio does help you lose weight, I've found that if you keep your focus on strength training, a moderate amount of cardio is adequate. So, don't spend hours on the treadmill! Simply do 20 to 30 minutes of fast-paced cardio 4 times a week, and that's enough. And keep things fast-paced because that way you'll burn more calories in a shorter amount of time.

My philosophy on weight training has always been that it's the one thing that'll keep your muscles strong and your bones healthy, and the more muscle you have, the more fat you'll burn. A quick way to gauge how to use weight training at any time during the year is to remember these guidelines: if I'm not training for a fight, I'll use heavier weights and fewer reps. When I'm back in the boxing gym training for a fight, I'll use lighter weights and lots of reps if I'm weight training. (For more on how to figure out the right size of weights for you, see the list in the section titled "My Favorite Weight-Training Exercises" below.)

My training regimen always changes. For example, I'll box in the morning or the evening. I might hit the weights four days a week. My cardio workouts could be doing the steps in Santa Monica or running. Everything I do is set up to mimic a ten-round fight, short and fast—a flurry of activity. Up those 187 steps and then resting for a minute on the way down. I do this 10 times in a row. That kind of boxing-workout mind-set can get you in great condition very quickly.

Cardio *First*, Then Weights

One of my workout philosophies has been to always start with cardio to ensure that I'm warmed up. As I get older, I feel this is a must.

If possible, I like doing all of my cardio outside, but if you can't, you can always use a treadmill or a stair climber. I stretch immediately after my cardio for about 20 minutes. I stretch only after I have broken a good sweat. When I hit that magical age of 40, I realized even more just how important stretching is for my body.

After my cardio warm-up, I'll start my weight training. I break this up into body parts: for example, shoulders, chest, and triceps on one day; the second day is back, biceps, and forearms; the third day is legs. I typically train my abs about 4 days a week when I'm not in training for a boxing match.

My Favorite Weight-Training Exercises

Over the years, I've found a number of weight-training exercises that work well for me. I've spent many hours in the gym and experienced a lot of frustration at times (we all want results *now!*) before I discovered the exercises that my body responds well to, but I finally found them. I've shown them to many people, and they have also gotten terrific results by using them. I know you will, too!

In a moment I'll describe them, but I want you to keep a few things in mind:

- You'll find that many exercises do not have a prescribed amount of weight you should use. Why? Because each of us is different in regard to fitness experience, strength, and level of expertise.
- To find the right weight for you, take time to experiment. If an exercise calls for 12 reps in a set, find the amount of weight that allows you to do 8 to 10 reps without too much difficulty but requires you to put some effort into completing those last few reps to reach 12.
- Once you are able to easily do 12 reps (for example) in an exercise, you're getting stronger, and now it's time to increase the weight by at least 10 percent. Follow that guideline for all of your weighted exercises.
- Never be afraid to experiment and change things around to make any exercise work well for you.

Regardless of what you may have heard or read all of these years, nothing about exercise or diet is set in stone. It's all open to change (changes that you will make!). You will tweak and revise each good exercise to make it a great one that's perfect for your body and your goals.

Now on to the exercises.

For the Shoulders

The shoulder muscles (delts) often don't get enough direct stimulation during the course of one's day, so to strengthen and shape this area I recommend the following exercises.

Mia's Move for the Delts: The Overhead Press

THE MOVE

You can use either a barbell or dumbbells. (For more on how to figure out the right size of weights for you, see the list above.) And let's dispel any fears and misconceptions. Strong and shapely shoulders look great! If women didn't want them, why would they buy dresses and tops with padded shoulders? If you do the overhead press, you won't need to use shoulder pads.

Many people have access to dumbbells or barbells at home, so it's not a requirement that you go to a gym to do either the dumbbell or the barbell version of the overhead press. Some people prefer to do these standing, others seated. Some people do them with a barbell, others with dumbbells. Certain individuals like to use a barbell and do them in front of the neck, while others like the feeling they get from using the barbell behind the neck. You may choose any variation you'd like. Keep the following tips in mind.

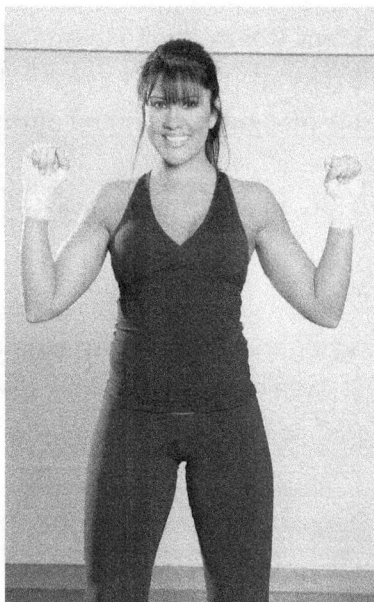

HOW TO DO IT

If you're using a barbell, take a slightly wider than shoulder width grip. Stand erect, with your feet about shoulder-width apart. Keep your head up as you look forward. Raise the weight up by extending your arms directly over your head. Now lower the bar behind your neck to the lower neck/upper traps area (or the upper-chest/clavicle area, if you prefer pressing from the front).

As you lower the weight, be sure to keep your elbows pointed down and not back. Keep your upper body in a vertically straight position throughout the movement. Take a deep breath in as you lower the weight, and exhale as you extend your arms and bring the weight back up above your head.

Quick tip: Using a nonstop motion will really make your delts burn, so do 2 to 3 sets of 8 to 12 nonstop reps each.

Mia's Move for the Delts: The Standing/Seated Dumbbell Side Lateral

THE MOVE

This is such a simple move. Stand straight up and raise your arms directly out to your sides to shoulder level, with your palms facing down. Did you do it? Great! You now know how to do a side lateral. Now let's do them with weights.

HOW TO DO IT

You have two choices for how you'd like to do this move: you can stand or sit. Your upper body will make the same movements for both variations of the

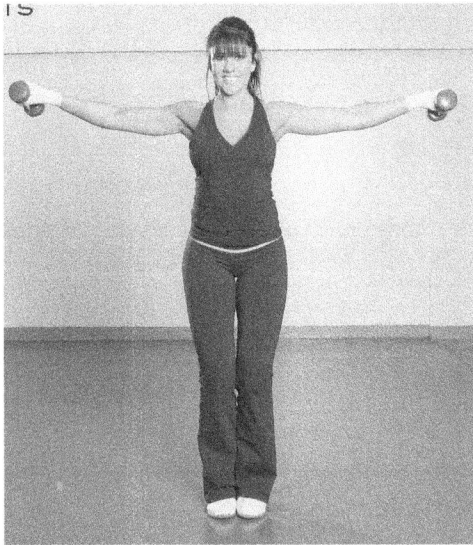

exercise. The only thing that changes is the placement of your lower body, sitting or standing.

For either exercise variation, you'll want your upper body to be vertically erect, straight up and down. Your head and neck are up as you look forward. Your abs are tight. Your arms will be fully extended downward, and you'll hold the dumbbells close to your sides, palms facing your legs, when you start the exercise. (For more on how to figure out the right size of weights for you, see the list in the section titled "My Favorite Weight-Training Exercises" in this chapter.)

From the bottom starting position, raise both arms up and directly out to your sides, away from your body. Make sure you raise your arms and the weights in a straight line, elbows not bent. Once your arms holding the dumbbells reach the top position at shoulder level, your palms will face the floor. Slowly lower your arms and the weights back down to the starting position (i.e., your arms extended straight down, with the weights hanging down against the outside of your thighs and your palms facing your thighs) again, and repeat. Many people find that if their arms go higher than shoulder level at the top of the move, they start to feel it more in the traps and less in the delts. Experiment and find the best stopping position for you.

Quick tip: The delts respond very well to nonstop high reps, so keep that in mind when you work them. Some people turn their wrists slightly forward (with the thumbs pointing toward the floor) once they reach the top of the exercise. Others say they don't feel any difference doing it like that. See which way feels best for you. Do 2 to 3 sets of 8 to 12 nonstop reps.

Mia's Move for the Delts: The Bent-Over Dumbbell Side Lateral Raise

THE MOVE

So, how did you like the dumbbell side lateral raise? It's a burner for sure, and it's one of those exercises where you can really see the muscles working as you do it.

Next, you'll do the bent-over dumbbell side lateral raise. This is a great exercise that will hit the rear head of the deltoid. You can do these moves standing or seated. The only difference between this exercise and the standing/seated dumbbell side laterals, which were described earlier, is the upper-body position. Instead of keeping the upper body upright and erect, you'll squat and bend forward until your head is over your feet and your upper torso is almost parallel to the floor.

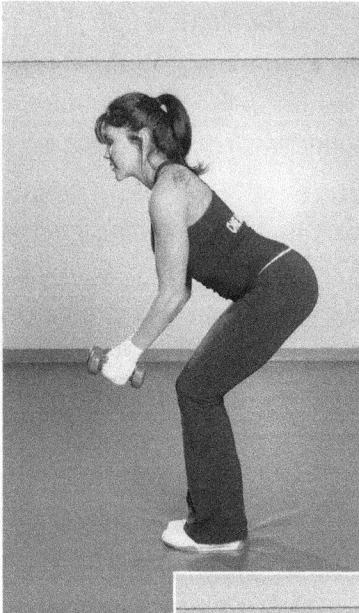

HOW TO DO IT

Think of this move as just like doing the side lateral, only this time your upper body will bend forward, either standing or seated (and will not be erect, as it was when you did the standing/seated side lateral). The arm motion will stay the same, but because your upper body is now bent over and forward, you will extend your arms down and in front of your body, holding the weights parallel and touching each other at about knee level, with your palms facing each other and your elbows slightly bent. From there, you'll simply bring your arms directly out to your sides until your hands and the weights are at shoulder level. Here are a few more helpful tips.

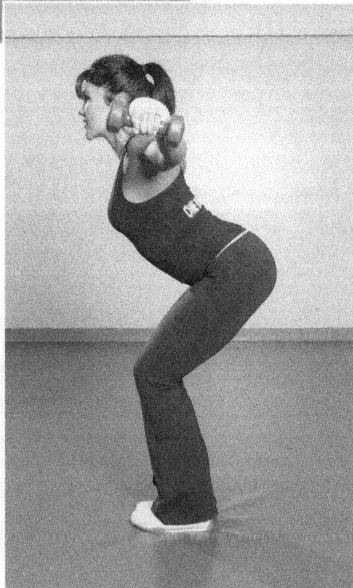

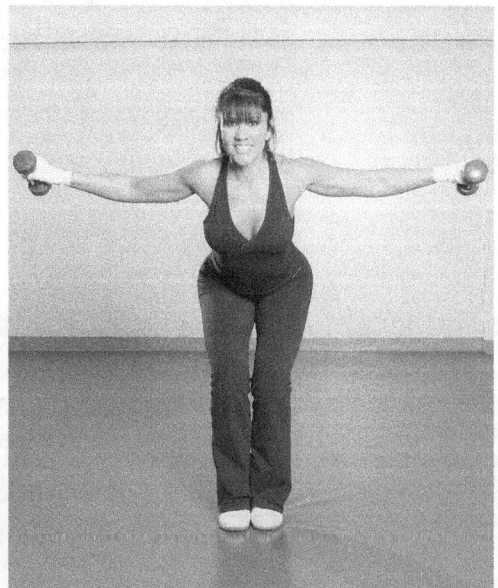

Inhale before you begin the exercise, then exhale as you raise your arms with the weights directly out to your sides. Inhale again as you lower your arms and the weights back to the starting position in front of your knees, with the insides of your wrists almost touching each other and the dumbbells parallel to each other. (For more on how to figure out the right size of weights for you, see the list in the section titled "My Favorite Weight-Training Exercises" in this chapter.)

Quick tip: Nonstop reps work great on all deltoid exercises, and this one is no exception. Don't allow the weights to stop at either the top or the starting position. Keep them moving! Do 2 to 3 sets of 8 to 12 nonstop reps.

Mia's Move for the Delts: The Uppercut with Dumbbells

THE MOVE

The uppercut is one of boxing's most powerful punches. It's typically executed when you and your opponent are face-to-face and so close that you're unable to reach your arms out with a jab or a straight punch. Your arms are tucked in close to your body, your palms face your body, and your knuckles face up toward the ceiling. The uppercut is when you bring your arm straight up toward the chin or the face of your opponent. Because your arm is so close to your upper body, you can generate a lot of power by using this punch. With that in mind, let's now put a dumbbell in each hand and make this a great move for your delts. (For more on how to figure out the right size of weights for you, see the list in the section titled "My Favorite Weight-Training Exercises" in this chapter.)

HOW TO DO IT

Get ready by placing your feet about shoulder width apart, with one foot forward and one foot back (whichever is most comfortable for you). Keep your knees slightly bent. Your abs will be tight and your upper body erect. Keep your neck and head up as you look forward. With a dumbbell in each hand (start with 2- to 5-pound dumbbells), first lift your right arm toward the ceiling as if punching a tall opponent under his or her chin. Be sure to lift until your arm is almost completely straight up and above you, but do not lock the elbow. Then bring the right arm back, tucked in close to your body, and do an uppercut with your left hand.

Quick tip: I like to turn my hips slightly into each lift and in the same direction as the lift. You will inhale before you begin, then exhale as you bring your arm with the weight up, and inhale as you lower the weight to the starting position. Do 2 to 3 sets of 8 to 12 nonstop reps for each side.

For the Chest

Besides having some of the biggest muscles in the body, the chest is an area that responds well to a multi-angle attack of working the upper, middle, and lower areas. Each person's body will respond to the same exercises differently.

Perhaps you'll find that dumbbells feel and work better, so you'll focus your chest work on using them. Or, maybe a combination of dumbbells, barbell, and machine feels best. The choice is yours. Here are the exercises.

Mia's Move for the Chest: Flat Bench Barbell Press

THE MOVE

This move is great for the overall chest. Many women want a great-looking chest and think it takes cosmetic surgery to get it. This is not so. You'll be pleasantly surprised at how much better your chest area will look once you start doing exercises that directly work the chest muscles that sit underneath the breasts.

You won't need to use heavy weights or do any exotic exercises. You'll stick with the tried-and-true basic moves, which will give you more strength and a shape you're sure to smile about. Here's the first exercise.

HOW TO DO IT

The flat bench barbell press is probably the most popular chest exercise that people do. Although it doesn't specifically target any specific chest region (i.e., upper, lower, outer, or inner chest), it does work the overall chest muscle (the pecs) in a good way. And it's a simple move.

To begin, lie down on your back on a flat bench. Take a slightly wider than shoulder-width grip on the barbell. (For more on how to figure out the right size of weights for you, see the list in the section titled "My Favorite Weight-Training Exercises" in this chapter.) As you look up, the barbell should be at about eye level. Lift the weight up and off the weight rack. Bring the weight slightly over your head and above your chest.

Take a deep breath in as you lower the weight and the bar to your lower chest area. You might have more power if you keep your elbows close to your sides while doing this exercise. Let the barbell touch the top of your chest. Now blow that deep breath out and begin to press the weight back up by fully extending your arms straight upward and the weight back up above your body.

Quick tip: If you want to feel the exercise work more of your upper chest, then bring the bar to your lower neck area and keep your elbows back to shoulder level. Do 2 to 3 sets, and stay in the range of 8 to 10 reps per set.

Mia's Move for the Chest: Incline Bench Press

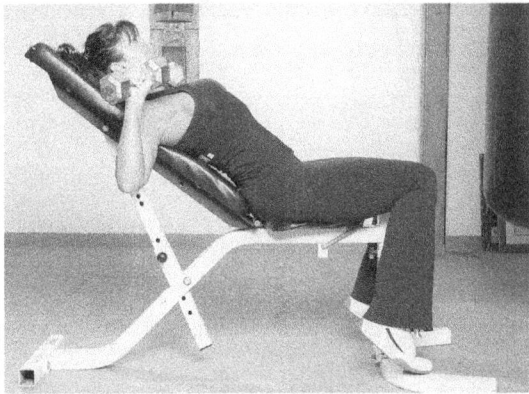

THE MOVE

This move is for the upper chest. This is similar to the flat bench press; however, you'll be using an incline bench instead of a flat bench. The incline bench will direct more of the chest work to your upper-chest area. (For more on how to figure out the right size of weights for you, see the list in the section titled "My Favorite Weight-Training Exercises" in this chapter.)

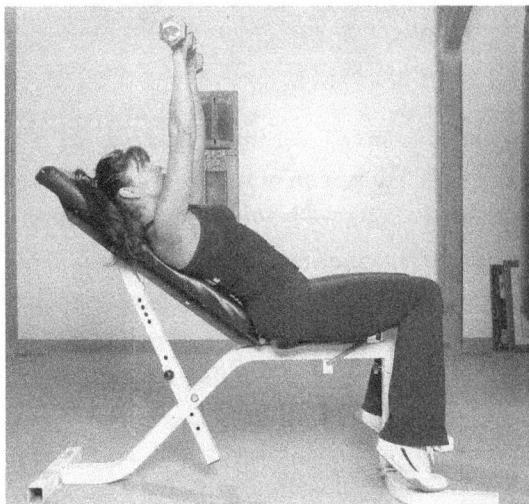

HOW TO DO IT

Begin the move by securely positioning your upper body on the bench. Keep your legs out in front of you, knees bent, and feet planted firmly on the floor. Take a medium grip on the bar with your hands about shoulder width apart. Take a deep breath and lock your arms out as you raise the weight up and off the weight rack.

Lift the weight high over your body until it's over your chin. Inhale and slowly lower the bar until it touches your upper body near your upper-chest/lower-neck area and inhale at the bottom position. Then exhale as you extend your arms and the weight back upward. Do 2 to 3 sets of 8 to 12 reps.

Quick tip: Try moving your hand position on the bar to feel it in different areas of your chest (i.e., place your hands closer together for more focus on the inner chest and your hands wider apart to focus on the outer chest).

Mia's Move: Close-Grip Bench Barbell Press

THE MOVE

This move is for the inner chest and the triceps. Remember how you did the flat bench press? Great, because you'll be using the same form, only this time your hands will be spaced about 6 to 8 inches apart on the barbell and not shoulder-width, as you did with the flat bench press. (For more on how to figure out the right size of weights for you, see the list in the section titled "My Favorite Weight-Training Exercises" in this chapter.) Here's a quick review.

HOW TO DO IT

To begin, lie down on a flat bench. Grip the bar so that your hands are fairly close together, no more than 6 to 8 inches apart. As you look up, the barbell should be about eye level. Lift the weight up and off the weight rack. Bring the weight slightly over your head and above your chest.

Take a deep breath in as you lower the weight and bar to your lower-chest area. You might have more power if you keep your elbows close to your sides

DID YOU KNOW THAT... There's a great all-natural stress and tension reliever that's ages old, yet very few people know about it. Mix together 1 teaspoon of sage leaves (known as nature's sleep helper), 1 tablespoon of rosemary leaves (known as nature's tranquilizer), and 1 ounce of dry peppermint leaves (known as nature's digestive). Keep the mixture in an airtight container (such as Tupperware). Boil some water and use 1 heaping teaspoon of the mixture to 1 cup of boiling water. Allow the mixture of leaves to sit for about 1 minute in the cup of hot water and strain the liquid into a fresh new cup. Add honey to sweeten it, and drink it with small sips. Talk about relaxing your mind and body "au naturel"!

while doing this exercise. Because your hands are so close together on the bar, it'll be hard for the bar to actually touch your chest, so just let it come down so that your hands touch the top of your chest. Now blow that deep breath out, and press the weight back up by extending your arms and the weight up above your body.

   Quick tip: Do 2 to 3 sets and, for a change, do higher reps in the 12 to 18 range.

Mia's Move for the Chest: Dumbbell Flys

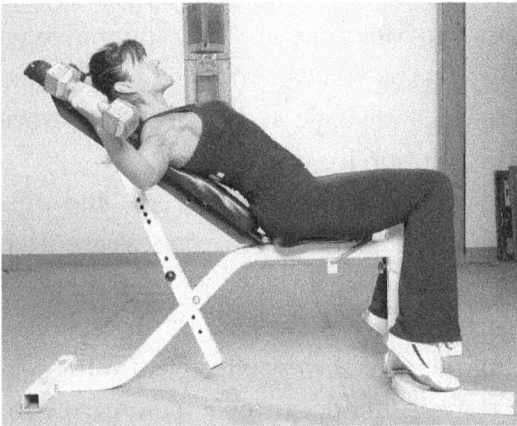

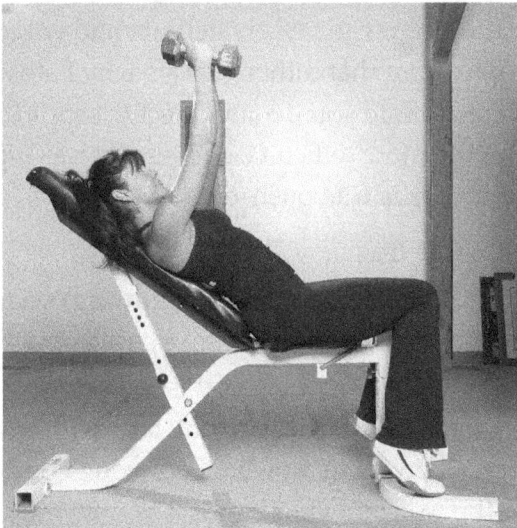

THE MOVE

Flys have got to be one of the best moves for shaping a great-looking chest. They're so easy to do—just think of putting your arms around a big barrel using a wide circular motion.

HOW TO DO IT

Lie on your back on a flat or slightly inclined bench and hold a dumbbell in each hand, with your arms out to your sides at shoulder level, elbows bent and palms facing upward. Place your feet flat on the floor in front of you. Keep your glutes and upper body resting firmly on the bench. Inhale.

   Exhale as you raise your arms above your upper body; keep your hands about 4 inches apart so that the dumbbells don't touch.

   Take a deep breath in as you bend your elbows slightly and as your arms and the weights come out and down to your sides at shoulder level. Your palms should face each other and the sides of your body as you lower your arms and the weights down to the bottom position.

You want to lower your arms and the dumbbells only far enough that you feel a good stretch, then, in a semicircular motion (just as if you were putting your arms around a big barrel), bring your arms and the weights back up until your arms are extended and your elbows locked and the weights are above your body. Repeat the sequence of moves. Do 2 to 3 sets with reps in the 8 to 12 range.

Quick tip: Try doing nonstop reps without locking your elbows. You'll really feel the chest burn, and that means you'll intensify the good results!

For the Triceps

Let's have a little fun. Stand in front of a mirror. Hold one arm up to about shoulder level, and bend your elbow so that your hand is higher than your shoulder and your arm looks like an "L." Now move your arm forward and backward as fast as you can and look at the muscle under your arm. Is it firm, or does it wiggle and jiggle? If it's moving and jiggling, then I've got the solution for you.

That muscle on the back of your arm is your triceps, and unless you're hitting it with exercises that target that area, chances are, it's not going to be as firm or toned as you'd like it to be.

I'm going to give you some great exercises for the triceps. Some will be easier than others, but they are all very effective. I want you to keep something very important in mind, however, before you work your triceps.

The triceps tendon near the elbow can be very delicate and vulnerable to injury, for some people more than others. That's why I always want you to warm up that area before you do any direct triceps exercises with weights or attempt the more difficult exercises, such as dips.

A great warm-up for the triceps is wall push-outs.

1. Stand about 1 to 2 feet away from a wall.
2. Place your hands (palms down, fingers pointing upward) on the wall in front of you, and make sure they are spaced roughly shoulder width apart.
3. While keeping your upper body in a straight line with your lower body, bend your elbows and slowly allow your body to come forward toward the wall and your hands.

4. As soon as your shoulders touch the backs of your hands, use only your arms/triceps to push your body back out to the starting position by straightening your arms until they are fully extended.

5. Do 1 or 2 sets of at least 8 to 12 reps per set.

Now you're ready for the exercises. I'll list them in the order of easiest to most difficult.

Mia's Move for the Triceps: The Triceps Kickback

THE MOVE

This is a great move because it is simple and doesn't require much weight, and simply changing the position of the exercising arm (i.e., keeping the elbow in line with the upper torso or raising it higher than the torso) increases the intensity of the exercise and of course, the result. So let's get right into it.

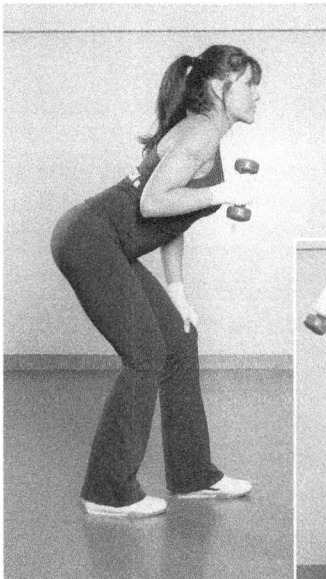

HOW TO DO IT

Let's practice this move without weights first. Stand up straight. Put your legs close together, with your left foot slightly ahead of the right. Bend your knees slightly. Let your upper body come forward so that your head is aligned over your front foot. Place your right arm against your upper body with your elbow bent so that your lower arm (forearm and hand) is below the upper in an "L" position. Place your left hand on your left knee for balance. While keeping your upper arm always firmly against (or close to) your upper body, extend your lower arm behind you and lock the elbow and arm out. That will be your peak contracted ending position. See, that was easy.

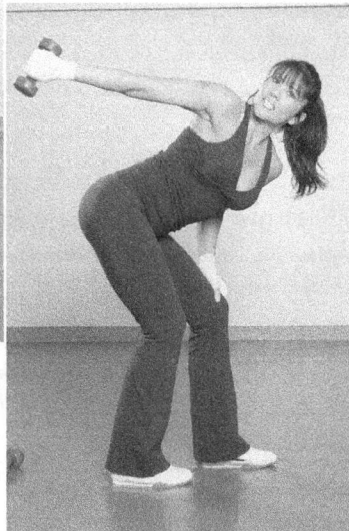

Now do 1 or 2 high-rep warm-up sets, just as I described and with either no weight (using only the weight of your arm) or a dumbbell with a very light weight for more than 15 reps. You want to increase blood flow to the triceps and elbow areas to make sure they are good and warmed up. After the warm-up, grab a dumbbell and add enough weight that'll allow you to do 6 to 10 reps per set. You will inhale before the exercise, then exhale while extending your arm out behind you to the contracted ending position. Then inhale as you lower your arm and bring the weight back to the starting position.

The big factor here is elbow position—you'll want to keep it slightly elevated and higher than your back, so that it will make your triceps work harder.

Do 20 reps for the warm-ups and 2 to 3 sets of 6 to 10 reps for the heavier sets.

Quick tip: When the dumbbell reaches the top of the movement, try turning your hand so that your palm is facing upward, which will contract the triceps even more.

Mia's Move for the Triceps: The Triceps Extension with Dumbbells

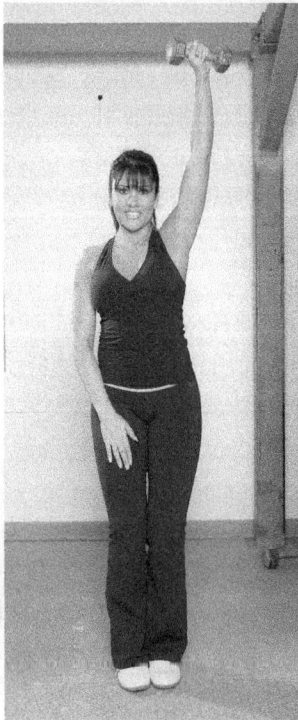

THE MOVE

You can do this standing or while sitting on a bench. For many people who've done triceps exercises only on machines, the triceps extension with dumbbells will be a move they'll immediately feel in their triceps in a whole new way. (For more on how to figure out the right size of weights for you, see the list in the section titled "My Favorite Weight-Training Exercises" in this chapter.) The key to this exercise is the position of the elbows. The more you can put your elbow in a position to make the triceps work harder, the more you'll feel it and the more effective the exercise will be. Here's how I like to do them.

HOW TO DO IT

Begin with the standing version. Grab a dumbbell with your left hand. Stand up straight, with your legs either locked or a slight bend in your knees (whichever you prefer). Keep your head and neck up and look straight in front of you. Your abs should be tight.

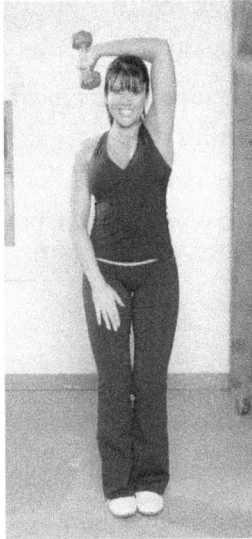

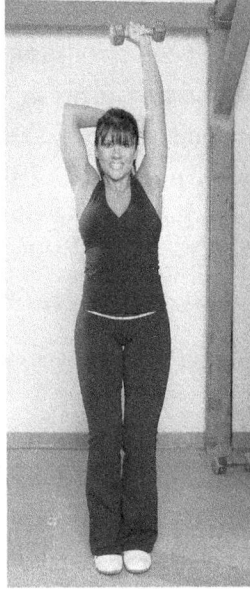

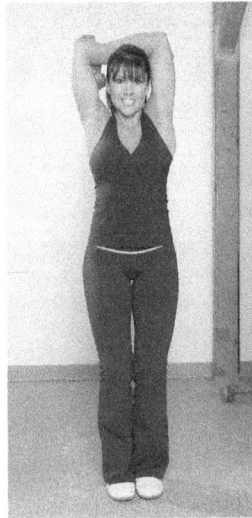

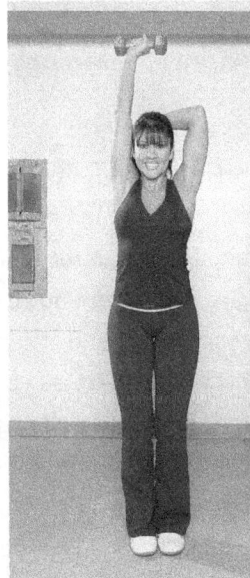

Now raise your left arm straight up so that the dumbbell's weight is directly overhead. You'll want your left arm to be in a vertical position with the upper arm nearly next to your head. Extend the arm with the dumbbell straight up until your elbow is locked and your palm is facing forward.

Bend your left elbow and allow your left hand holding the dumbbell to come down behind your head, while your left upper arm stays vertical beside your head. You have four choices of position for the nonworking arm: place your nonworking hand on the front of your thighs, fingers pointing down; use the nonworking hand to hold onto an immovable object for support; keep the nonworking arm straight up but with the elbow bent, the upper arm beside your head, and the nonworking hand grabbing the elbow of the arm that's holding the dumbbell; or place the nonworking hand across your chest, holding the opposite side of your body. Do 10 to 15 reps, and then repeat with your right hand holding the dumbbell.

For the bench version of this move, you'll use two dumbbells at the same time, instead of one as you used for the standing version. Simply lie down on a flat bench. Raise your legs up off the bench, extended straight out, and cross your feet at the ankles. The higher up your legs are, the easier it will be. You can also bend your legs at a 90-degree angle. To make this exercise more challenging, lower your legs until they are only 1 or 2 feet above the bench. Your head, shoulders, back, and glutes should be the only body parts touching the bench.

Holding a dumbbell in each hand, bring your upper arms back and toward your head at about a 45-degree angle. Keep your elbows in that position and lower the weight. Now extend your arms straight upward with the elbows locked. Inhale as you lower your arms and the weights, and exhale as you raise your arms and the weights back up to the fully extended position.

Quick tip: Doing more reps in the 14 to 20 range works great for this move. Do 2 to 3 sets for either the standing triceps extension or the bench version.

Mia's Move for the Triceps: Dips

THE MOVE
Earlier, you did this move using a bench or a chair. The mechanics of this move (i.e., using your upper arms to raise and lower your body) will be similar. The difference is that you'll use a dip bar on a machine, and you won't be in the seated position while performing the exercise. Your body will be free, with only your arms doing the work. You'll need access to a dip bar to do it, and if you have one, then you really should give this exercise a go. You'll find dips to be one of the best lower-chest/triceps exercises you can do.

HOW TO DO IT
The key to making this exercise very effective is keeping your upper body fairly upright and your arms close to your sides from start to finish. You can either let your legs hang straight down underneath your upper body or bend your knees so that your feet are up and behind you.

Enter the dip bar. Take an equal overhand grip on each side of the bar. Keep your upper body erect, with your head up as you look forward. Keep your upper arms close to your upper body. Now allow your elbows to bend as you lower your body. Go as far down as is comfortably possible. Once you reach the bottom position, raise your body up until your arms are straight, with the elbows in the fully locked position. Inhale as you lower your body, and exhale as you bring it up to the starting position.

At first, you may not be able to do more than a few reps, but that's okay. Just go for as many reps as you can do. I've found that when I vary the distance of how far I bring my body down, I feel it in different ways. For example, on a few reps you might try coming all the way down as far as comfortably possible. For the next few reps, try coming only halfway down. Then for a few more reps, try doing partial reps by allowing a slight bend at the elbows and letting the upper body come down just a few inches. Best of all, mix it up: do a set in which you combine all three moves.

Start out by doing these only with your body weight, and once it gets easy to do 12 to 15 reps this way, then add weight plates or a dumbbell by using a dipping belt and a chain (to hold the weight plates or the dumbbell between your legs). Go for 2 to 3 sets. As you would with all triceps exercises, be sure to always do a really good warm-up (especially for the elbows) before doing dips.

Quick tip: Here are a couple of other ways you can do regular dips:

- With your arms/hands farther apart or closer together, if your dip bar is shaped like a V, with the wide part of the V at one end of the dip bar and the narrow part of the V at the other end.
- The V-shaped dip bar works great because it allows you to isolate other muscles better than the even-spaced dip bars will.
- Do dips with your hands closer together at the narrowest part of the V to work your triceps more.
- Do dips with hands farther apart at the widest part of the V to work your chest muscles more.
- How you position your elbows—either in and close to your upper body or out and away from your body—will also cause different feelings in your muscles.
- Do dips with your legs hanging straight down and in line with your upper body, provided that your dip bar is high enough off the floor to allow your body to come all the way down—with your legs straight—when you reach the bottom of the dip position with your elbows bent.
- Do dips with your knees bent and your lower legs and feet behind your body.

Mia's Move for Triceps: The Bench Dip

THE MOVE

This move is much like the triceps dips I told you about on page 148. I've found this to be a super exercise for adding size and shape to the lower triceps, the area above the elbow that typically doesn't get a lot of direct work. Be sure to do a warm-up for your triceps first.

HOW TO DO IT

To begin, you'll need a flat bench to place your hands on and either another bench or a chair about 3 to 4 feet away from you, to place your heels on.

Put your body in a position as if you are creating a body bridge; your feet are in front of you, resting on the bench or the chair (you can even bend your knees slightly if you'd like) and your hands/arms are holding your body up off the ground.

You'll want to keep your upper body as erect as possible. Keep your neck and head up as you look forward and your abs tight. Hold your upper arms in and close to your upper body from start to finish. Your elbows should always point behind you.

Start with your arms locked and fully extended, then bend your elbows and slowly let your body come down as far as is comfortably possible. After you reach the bottom position of the move, bring your body back up by straightening your arms. Inhale as you lower your body, and exhale as you bring it back up.

Quick tip: Do nonstop continuous reps until you've either done all that you can or you've performed 15 to 20. If you've done 15 to 20 reps and they were easy, then try putting a weight plate on top of your lap to give your body a little extra weighted resistance. Do 2 to 3 sets.

For the Biceps

A lot of people think of the upper arm as the biceps, but actually your upper arm has two muscles: the triceps (the three muscles in the back of the arm) and the biceps (the two muscles of the front or the top of the arm).

In many gyms, I've seen women doing biceps curls with very light weights, and then they wonder why they don't get any results. One reason is that they aren't using enough weight to cause the biceps to work harder and, in return, become stronger and better conditioned.

Many women are afraid that if they use heavier weights, they'll get too big and muscle-bound, and to that I say, "You have nothing to worry about." If people only knew how hard it is to put on muscle and how much weight they would need to lift and how many times they would have to do it, it would change all of their preconceived ideas about lifting weights.

Whether it's for the biceps, the triceps, the chest, or any other muscle, your body will respond better if you include *some* heavier-weight workouts in your exercise program. Muscle is healthy. Muscle is living tissue that needs calories. (Hint: With more muscle, you can eat more, weigh less, and look great.) Muscle changes the shape of your body and sculpts it to look better. Muscle keeps you strong and conditioned. Don't be afraid to have a little more muscle.

I'm going to give you some of the best barbell and dumbbell exercises to do, either at home or in a gym. These exercises work superbly anywhere.

Before you begin an exercise for any body part, always be sure to warm up. I suggest that for each exercise, do a warm-up of 1 or 2 sets of that exercise with light weights to get your blood flowing and muscles working before you jump into your normal weight training. Always use great form for every exercise.

Mia's Move for the Biceps: The Standing Dumbbell/Barbell Curl

THE MOVE

The dumbbell/barbell curl is one of the most basic biceps exercises you can do. The majority of people who train with weights have done them at one time or another in their workouts and for good reason: they work!

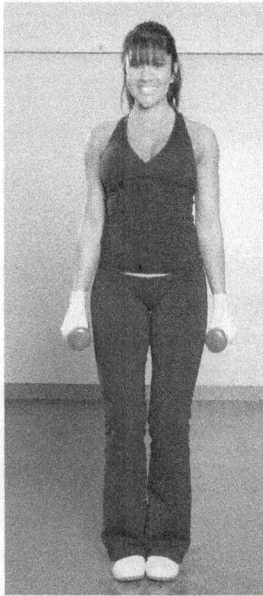

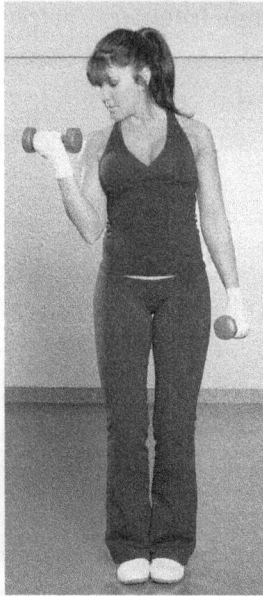

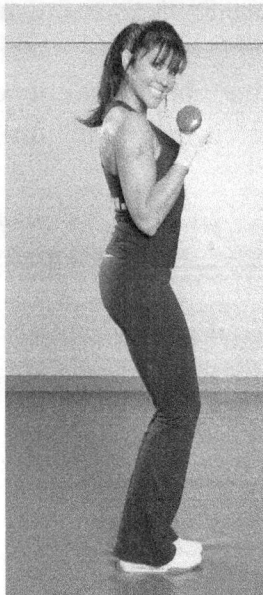

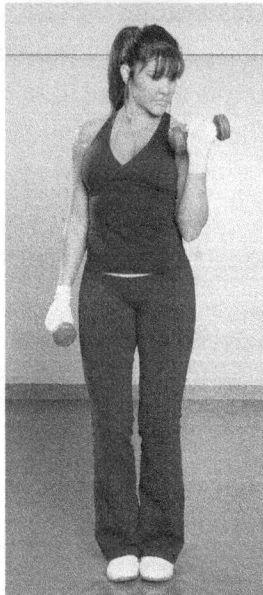

The key to making any biceps curl effective is twofold: the stretch at the bottom of the movement and the contraction at the top. When many people do these curls, they don't allow their arms and the weights to return to the fully extended starting position, with their arms straight down at their sides, and they curl the weights up too high and too far back, thereby allowing the biceps to decrease its contraction. (For more on how to figure out the right size of weights for you, see the list in the section titled "My Favorite Weight-Training Exercises" in this chapter.) Here's how I want you to do them.

HOW TO DO IT

Begin by standing erect with your feet about shoulder-width apart or a comfortable width for you and with your toes pointing forward. If you want to bend your knees slightly, that's okay. Keep your upper body erect, your neck and head up as you look forward. Keep your abs tight.

Allow the weights to hang down to your upper thighs as your arms are extended straight downward. Curl the weight in your right hand up to about chest level or the point where you feel your biceps fully contract. Hold this position for a count and then slowly lower the weight back down to the starting position. Inhale before you begin the exercise, exhale as you curl the weight up, and inhale as you lower the weight back to the starting position. Then do the same movement with your left arm holding the dumbbell. Reps in the 5 to 9 range work well. Do 2 to 3 sets.

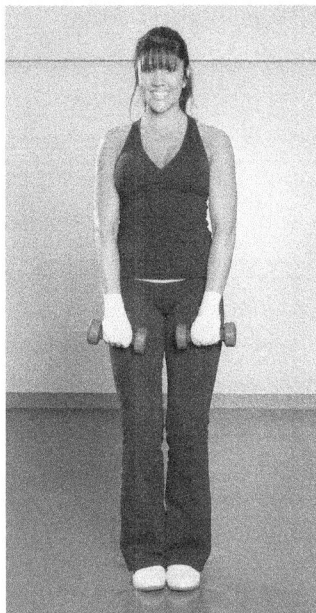

THE MOVE

When people think of arms that are in shape, they immediately think of the biceps. Biceps are the visual muscle. Just hold your arm up, flex it and "make a muscle," and boom! You see the biceps.

But did you know that the biceps is only about one-third of the muscle mass that makes up your arm size? The triceps (that three-headed muscle in the back of your arm) comprises the other two-thirds of your arm size.

We use our biceps every day when we pick up things. Yet while we may use those biceps for daily tasks, we rarely give them the kind of direct work they need to become stronger and more shapely.

Here's a move that's about to change that. Think of doing it like you would a regular dumbbell curl; however, you'll be changing the position of your hands during the exercise.

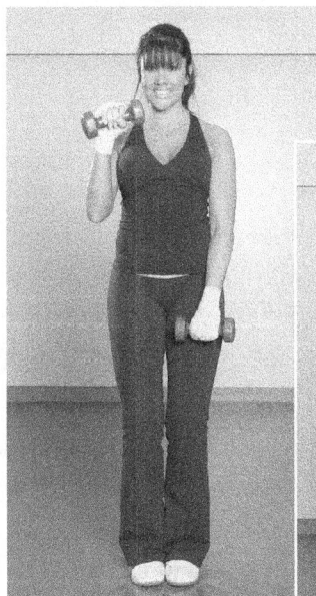

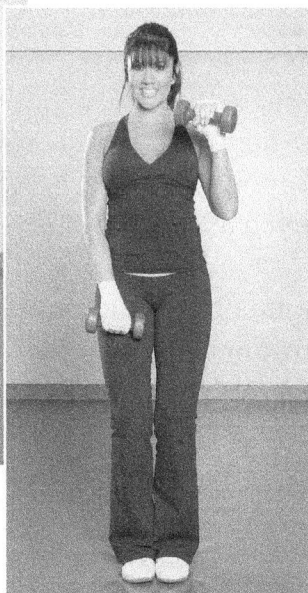

HOW TO DO IT

As the name says, you'll do these with dumbbells (one in each hand), standing erect, and in the ending position your palms will be up and facing out in front of you. (For more on how to figure out the right size of weights for you, see the list in the section titled "My Favorite Weight-Training Exercises" in this chapter.)

The move is simple. Stand with your body straight and your feet together or shoulder width apart. Keep your head up as you look forward. Keep both upper arms close to the sides of your body as your arms hang straight down, with a dumbbell in each hand. Your palms are facing in toward your thighs.

Take a deep breath, then slowly exhale as you begin to curl the dumbbell in your right hand by bringing only your right forearm and hand up to about shoulder level or to the point where you feel a peak biceps contraction. If you curl the weight up too high and let the upper arm and the dumbbell come back too close to the shoulder, you'll go past the point of peak contraction, which is the position where the exercise is most effective. Only the right forearm, the hand, and the weight should move upward as you curl the weight, while your upper arms stay locked next to the sides of your upper body.

Once you have reached the top of the movement with the biceps in a peak contraction position, slowly lower the weight back down to the starting position. Take a deep breath when you reach the bottom position, then exhale as you switch sides and begin to curl the dumbbell in your left hand following the same instructions. Repeat for a total of 10 to 12 alternating reps for each arm.

Rest no longer than 45 seconds and begin your next set. Do a total of 2 to 3 sets of 10 to 12 reps each.

Quick tip: Bring the weight up and stop once your palm faces the ceiling at the top of the move. If your palm faces behind you, you've gone too far.

For the Forearms

I'd be willing to bet that you probably couldn't tell me when you last did a forearm exercise. Maybe never? Don't feel bad. Most women haven't. But you're about to change all of that and for good reason.

Think about how important your forearms are for the actions you perform each day. Anytime you pick up an object and hold it in your grip, you're using your forearm.

I've found that not only did having well-conditioned forearms help me in every physical activity I undertook, be it boxing, weight training, or other sports, but my forearms made my entire body more aesthetically pleasing. Don't worry, you won't turn into Popeye by doing these exercises, either.

THE MOVE

This move is good for both the biceps and the forearms. I've found an easy way for you to remember how to work the forearms. Use the exact same form you did for the standing barbell curl, only this time place your hands in an overhand grip on the bar instead of the underhand grip that you used on the regular biceps barbell curl. If you're using dumbbells, simply use the same overhand grip throughout the exercise by keeping your palms facing the floor from start to finish. (For more on how to figure out the right size of weights for you, see the list in the section titled "My Favorite Weight-Training Exercises" in this chapter.)

HOW TO DO IT

If you are using a barbell, begin by taking a slightly wider than shoulder-width grip on the bar. Stand erect with your feet about shoulder-width apart and your toes pointing forward. If you want to bend your knees slightly, that's okay. Keep your upper body erect, and your neck and head up as you look forward. Keep your abs tight.

Bring your elbows in and close to the sides of your body, and keep your elbows locked to your sides from start to finish. Allow the weight to hang down to your upper thighs, with your arms extended straight down.

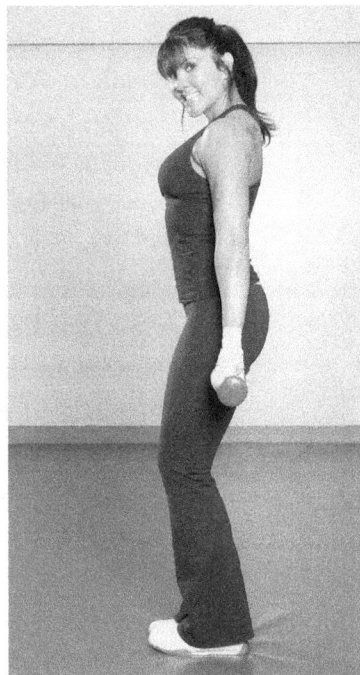

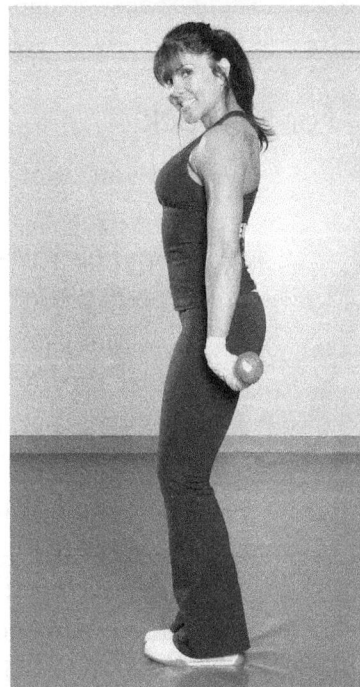

Curl the weight up to about mid-chest level or the point where you feel your forearms fully contracted. Hold for a count and then slowly lower the weight back down to the starting position. Your breathing will be: inhale before you begin the exercise, exhale as you curl the weight up, and inhale as you lower the weight back to the starting position.

Quick tip: Holding the bar in the fully contracted upright position for 3 to 5 seconds will really make those forearms burn. High reps in the 12 to 20 range work well. Do 2 to 3 sets.

If you are using dumbbells, stand erect with your feet about shoulder-width apart and your toes pointing forward. If you want to bend your knees slightly, that's okay. Keep your upper body erect, and your neck and head up as you look forward. Keep your abs tight.

Holding a dumbbell in each hand, bring your arms in close to the sides of your body and keep your elbows locked from start to finish. Allow the weights to hang down to your upper thighs, with your arms extended straight down and your palms facing down and backward.

Without moving your arms, rotate your wrists backward to bring each dumbbell up slightly behind your hands. Rotate the wrists forward again to bring the dumbbells forward and closer to the floor. Repeat this forward and backward movement for 2 to 3 sets of 15 to 20 reps each.

For the Back

If you want to look good, be more active, and help keep your body injury-free, it's essential to have a strong and well-conditioned back. Your back is a pillar in the center of your body, a foundation that supports you.

Many people make the mistake of doing lots of ab work, thinking that they are working the core muscles the way these need to be worked, but unless they are doing equal amounts of work for the back, they can run into major problems.

Think of the stomach and the back as opposite twins, with one always trying to pull against the other. Too much ab work and not enough back work can lead to an imbalance in function. Conversely, too much back work and not enough ab work can lead to problems, too. The key is to do equal amounts of work for both areas. I've found that it's best to do both ab and back work on the same day during the same workout.

Just as you can target many areas of the other muscles, you can do so with the back. You can start at the top of the back with the traps (trapezius muscles), move down to the Teres major, Teres minor, and Infraspinatus muscles near the shoulders, and then to the lats (the outer muscle that gives the body a V-tapered look) and the erectors (the muscles on both sides of the spine that run from the glutes on up).

We all like to train the body parts that we can easily see in the mirror, but to have a complete and balanced body and structure, we also need to train the body parts that are less visible, such as the lower back, the glutes, and the hamstrings. Don't worry, I've got you covered with these. Here are some of my favorite back exercises.

Mia's Move for the Back: The Dumbbell Row

THE MOVE

I like using dumbbells because they allow a greater range of motion than barbells or machines do. (For more on how to figure out the right size of weights for you, see the list in the section titled "My Favorite Weight-Training Exercises" in this chapter.) For your back, this exercise will give you a greater range of motion and help you better work the lats. I suggest doing dumbbell rows with one knee up off the floor and positioned on a flat bench and your opposite leg slightly bent with your foot firmly planted on the floor or atop an elevated platform. You can also do these standing with your upper body bent forward and with a slight bend to the knees.

HOW TO DO IT

To begin, take a dumbbell in your right hand. Place your left knee up on the bench and off the floor. Bend your right leg slightly and angle it out to your side, with your right foot firmly planted on the floor. Bend your upper body forward. Place your left arm on top of the bench for support.

With the dumbbell in your right hand, lower the weight as far down as possible to stretch your lats. Go for the fully extended right arm position. Once you reach the bottom, bring your elbow back and the weight up until your right hand is even with the side of your upper torso. Inhale as you lower the weight and exhale as you bring your arm with the weight back up.

Then repeat these movements for the other side, using a dumbbell in your left hand and reversing the positions of your legs on the bench and the ground.

Quick tip: The goal is to go for the fully extended arm position, causing the lat stretch at the bottom and the peak contraction at the top of the move. So, do it slowly until you're able to achieve that; however, keep your shoulder stabilized by not allowing it to hyper-extend. Reps in the 6 to 10 range work well. Go for 2 to 3 sets on each side.

Mia's Move for the Back: The Seated Cable Row

THE MOVE

Seated cable rows are a terrific move that not only works the back and the lats, but helps increase your range of motion all at the same time. You will need access to a seated cable row machine. This is a machine found in most health clubs that has a long low bench where you sit facing the weight stack, with foot pads to position your feet against and a cable and handle that runs between your legs. You can use many different types of bar attachments for this move, but the one I like is the stirrup-style bar. Here's how I want you to do them.

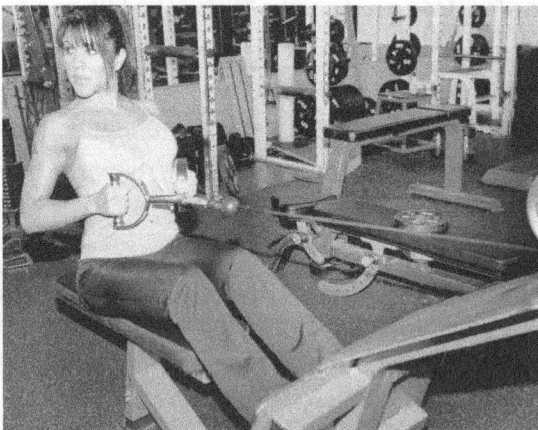

HOW TO DO IT

Use a stirrup-style bar so that your palms face each other. Grab the bar, position your body back on the bench, and plant your feet firmly on the foot platform.

Slightly bend your knees and keep your upper torso erect, with your neck and head up as you look forward. Keep your abs tight.

Let your arms and the bar extend fully in front of you. Then, with your upper body

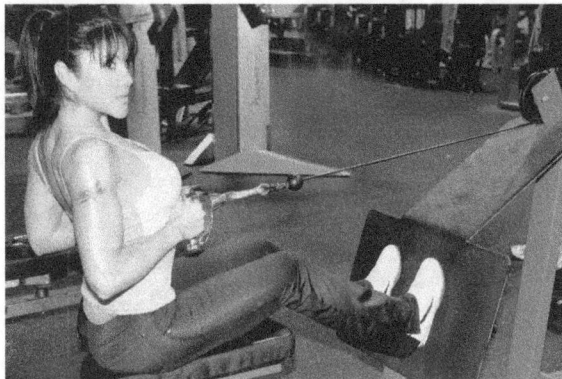

still erect, pull your elbows back behind you and the bar down low and back until your hands touch your lower stomach area just above the waist. This will be the peak contracted position of the move.

Next, lower the weight by bringing the bar and your arms forward to the fully extended position again, which is the starting position. Inhale before the exercise, exhale as you bring the bar and your arms back, and inhale as you return the bar and your arms to the starting position.

Quick tip: Allow your upper torso to come only slightly forward for a good lat stretch. Try for 8 to 12 reps and 2 to 3 sets.

Mia's Move for the Lower Back, the Glutes, and the Hamstrings: The Barbell/Dumbbell Dead Lift

THE MOVE

This is a truly great exercise for your hamstrings and lower back—and it's easy to do. Think of squatting down and then coming back up. We'll add a few more specifics, but that's essentially the gist of it. To get the most from this exercise, you need to really stretch. So if your range of motion isn't limited, you might want to stand on a wooden platform that's about 4 to 6 inches high so you can get an even greater stretch.

HOW TO DO IT

Begin the exercise by holding the dumbbells down at your sides. (For more on how to figure out the right size of weights for you, see the list in the section titled "My Favorite Weight-Training Exercises" in this chapter.) Stand with your upper body erect and slightly bend the knees. Keep your abs tight and your neck and head up as you look forward.

Now allow your upper torso to bend forward, with your head over your feet. As you lower your arms and the weights, rotate the dumbbells forward so that they are in front of your shins and your palms face back toward your body. Be sure to keep the weights close to your legs.

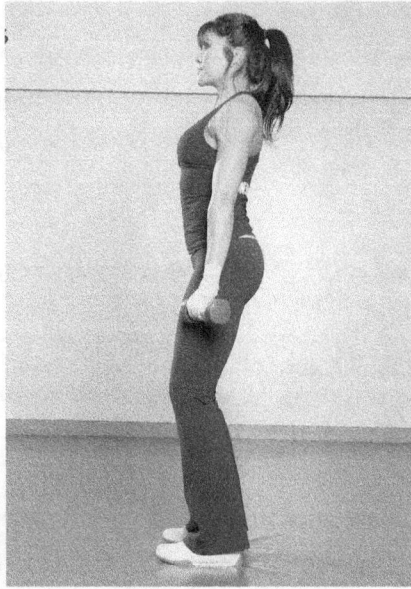

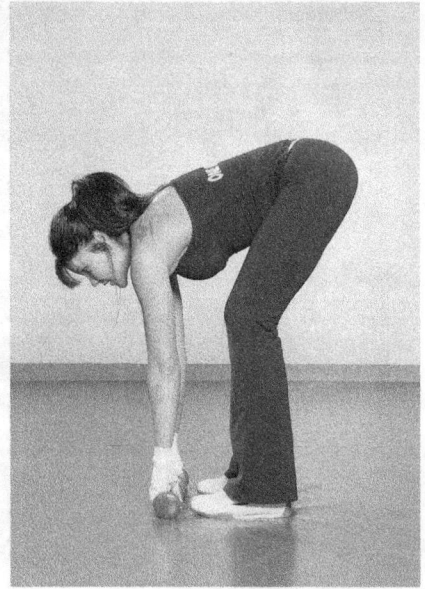

Also, keep your back slightly arched with your head up and in line with your upper back. You can keep your knees either locked or slightly bent, depending on which feels best to you. Go as far down as you can to feel that your hamstrings are fully stretched and then come back up to the starting position. Inhale as you lower your arms with the weights, and exhale as you bring the weights back up to the starting position. Do 6 to 8 reps per set and 2 to 3 sets.

Quick tip: Some people will be able to go down only to calf level. Others may stop a little higher, and some will bend so far down that the weights are below their feet (if they're using a platform).

Mia's Move for the Back: The Machine Lat Pulldown— to the Front of the Body

THE MOVE

Over the years, lat pulldowns and chin-ups have helped many, many guys widen out and achieve that V-look, with a wide upper torso and lats that spread out under the arms and taper down to a narrow waist. As eight-time Mr. Olympia Lee Haney once told Robert Wolff, "It's one thing to do a lat pulldown, but there's nothing like pulling your whole body up and down like a chin-up." Absolutely.

Chin-ups can be tough, and they will produce great results; however, not all women can do them or many reps of them. That's why I recommend machine lat pulldowns.

You'll need access to a lat pulldown machine, and these can be found at almost any health club or gym. You'll have lots of choices for how you do pulldowns, ranging from using a straight bar with a wide, medium, or close grip hand spacing, to doing them in front of your body or behind your neck. You can also choose what kind of bars or handle attachments to use. I like using a V-shape handle and doing pulldowns to the front of my body. The choice is yours.

HOW TO DO IT

As with all exercises, proper form is important not only to prevent injury, but to maximize the effectiveness of the exercise.

Begin by grabbing the bar/V-handle and sit down so that the front of your upper body is in a straight line under the high pulley of the machine just above your head. Keep your upper body erect and your neck and head up as you look forward. Keep your abs tight.

With a slight arch to your back so that your upper torso is now slightly forward, pull the bar/handle down and let it touch the top of your upper-chest area. As you pull the bar/handle down, focus on bringing your elbows down, back, and behind you, as this will help give you a better lat/back contraction.

In a controlled movement, allow the bar/handle and your arms to come back up and return to the starting position. Continue this sequence until you've completed all of the reps in your set. Do 2 to 3 sets of 10 to 15 reps.

A breathing reminder: you'll find it helpful to take a deep breath before you begin each rep and then, as you start the rep, breathe out while you pull the bar down and your arms back. As you reach the full-contraction stage of the rep (i.e., when the bar/handle hits the top of your chest area), inhale as your arms come back up and return to the starting position.

Quick tip: An easy way to remember how to breathe for all of your exercises is to take a deep breath in before you begin the exercise, use an even, controlled exhalation as you reach the first half of the exercise (the contraction), and then take another deep breath in (the inhalation) as you return the weight and your body to the starting position for that exercise.

For the Legs

It seems that so many people want great-looking legs but don't want to put in the time or effort to create them. Unless you're genetically gifted, you simply won't have the legs you want unless you do the exercises that will shape them.

I've found that working the legs is probably one of the hardest, if not *the* hardest, body part that I train. To do it right, it takes a lot of energy. During a good leg workout, there'll be many times when you'll feel like quitting, but don't you dare! *That's* the point when you know you're making progress and making your legs work hard enough to quickly change their shape, conditioning, and appearance.

The hamstrings are one of those muscles that, for most people, never get any direct work from specially targeted exercises. Just like the abs-to-back relationship of push/pull, protagonist/antagonist, if you have strong front leg muscles and weak back leg muscles, you're setting yourself up for getting injured down the road.

I don't want that to happen and I know you don't either, so here are some excellent hamstring (back of the leg) exercises that will promote good leg muscle balance.

Women love to have awesome calves. Although it's nice to have killer legs (or "gams," as they used to say years ago), people immediately notice a great set of calves, especially when you're wearing a dress and heels.

First, here are some of my favorite front of the leg (quad) exercises.

Mia's Moves for the Fronts of the Legs (Quads): The Squat (see "The Squat" on page 125)

THE MOVE

One of the best exercises you can do for your legs is the squat. This exercise not only targets the front leg muscles (the quads), but also works the hamstrings, the glutes, and the lower back at the same time. Proper form is essential when performing the squat. You want your upper body to be erect, your head up as you look forward, and your upper leg to stop about parallel to the floor when you reach the bottom of the movement. Be sure to keep your knees in line with your toes, and do not let your knees go forward past the toes at the bottom position. Squats can be tough, but they are a great leg exercise, indeed!

HOW TO DO IT

Stand erect, with your head up as you look forward, and place your feet about shoulder width apart and pointing in front of you. Keep your abdominals pulled in. Bring your arms out in front of your body. Cross your arms so your hands rest on opposite elbows. While keeping your arms out in front of you, shift your weight back onto your heels, inhale, and bend your knees as you squat down. (Pretend there's a chair behind you and you're about to sit in it as you lower yourself into a squatting position.) Go no lower than having your upper legs parallel to the floor. Stopping a little higher than parallel is just fine.

As you get ready to return to the top starting position, squeeze your glutes and exhale as you bring your body up. Keep your chest lifted from start to finish, and don't sit lower than the upper-legs-parallel-to-floor point or let your knees go forward past your toes. Go for 2 to 3 sets of 12 to 15 reps each.

If you're doing back squats with a barbell and weights, let the bar rest high on your upper-back/shoulder area somewhere on the traps. Take a grip on each side of the bar that's slightly wider than your shoulders. Place your feet about shoulder-width apart and turn them slightly out. For more stability, you may want to slightly elevate your heels an inch or two. Using two weight plates works great as a heel raise.

Use the same exercise form that was just described, but add a slight arch to your lower back and keep your head up and looking straight ahead. Squat down until your thighs are about parallel to the floor. Always make sure your knees travel in a direct line over your big toes.

You will inhale before bending your knees and lowering the weight as you reach the bottom position; then exhale as you bring your body and the weight up to the starting position. Do 2 to 3 sets of 8 to12 reps.

Quick tip: For variety and to work the inner thighs, try doing wide-stance squats. Essentially, you'll do them the same way you just did the regular squat, using the same upper-body positioning. The only difference is the placement of your feet. To work your inner thighs, you'll keep your legs and feet about 2 to 3 feet apart and turn your feet outward (always making sure when you squat that your knees align with the big toes, but don't go forward past the toes). Higher reps in the 12 to 16 range work well. Do 2 to 3 sets.

Mia's Move for the Legs: The Leg Extension

THE MOVE

This is a good exercise to warm up the knee area and the quads. High nonstop reps (more than 15) work great on leg extensions. The main thing to remember is to feel the quads working as you do this. Some people will use their full range of motion and do continuous reps. Others will use a combination of full-range reps and then partial reps, allowing their feet to come down only a few inches before extending their legs again, locking their legs out, and squeezing the quads for 1 to 2 seconds before doing the next rep. You will need access to a leg extension machine.

HOW TO DO IT

Be sure your body is positioned back far enough so that the area where your hamstrings and calves meet is touching the seat. Keep your upper body erect and your back against the seat back pad. Your neck and head will be up as you look forward. Keep your abs tight.

Begin the move by bringing the pad/your lower legs up until you reach the lock-out position at the top of the exercise. Hold this for a count, and then slowly lower the pad/your lower legs back down to the starting position.

Go for the full quad stretch by having your feet come back as far as possible under the seat at the bottom of the exercise. You'll find that nonstop high reps work great. Inhale before beginning the exercise, exhale as you bring your lower legs up and contract the quads, and inhale as you lower the pad/your lower legs back to the starting position.

Quick tip: You might want to try doing a set with your feet pointed forward, another set with your feet turned inward and pointed toward each other, and a third set with them turned outward. Some people swear by this because they say they feel it in different areas of the quads. Go for reps in the 15 to 25 range. Do 2 to 3 sets.

Mia's Move for the Legs: The Lunge and the Walking Lunge
(see "The Walking Lunge" on page 126)

THE MOVE

I'm sure you've seen people do lunges, but many do them incorrectly despite using the right form, because they do them with so little intensity that the lunges produce no noticeable results.

The trick is to use great form but make your quads burn by doing nonstop reps. That means no resting at the top of the exercise for a second or two and then going down again. I want you doing nonstop reps and to do all of the reps for the set for each leg before you change legs.

Be sure to keep your knee in a direct line over your big toe during the exercise to prevent injury. I suggest going down far enough that your upper leg is lower than parallel to the floor. I think you'll feel the exercise more. Always keep the quad of your nonworking leg in a direct line with your upper torso and not in front or behind. You can either hold the dumbbells down at your sides or up next to your shoulders, as if you are doing a press. Keep your palms facing your cheeks.

HOW TO DO IT

The walking lunge is one of my favorite exercises to target not only the fronts and the backs of the legs, but the glutes as well. I see many women doing lunges, but very few do them correctly. Or perhaps I should say, "effectively." As with any exercise, it's easy to just go through the motions, but that's not what you want to do. You want results, and you'll get them by focusing directly on the muscles and using great form. The good news is, you don't even need to use weights (your body weight alone will do) to get terrific results.

Begin by standing up straight with your legs and feet together. Keep your chest raised, your upper body erect, your back straight, and your abdominals pulled in, while your head looks forward. With your right foot, take a large step forward. Now drop your left knee down toward the ground, and try to keep it directly under your body and in as close a direct line with your upper body as you can. Be sure to keep your upper body upright and facing forward while you're at the bottom position.

Now bring your upper body up and move your left leg forward and bring your right leg down, directly under your body, with the right knee touching the floor, and repeat the same exercise sequence.

Quick tip: Keep moving forward (one leg, then the other) until you reach the end of the room or someplace where you can turn around and repeat the lunges for your next set. You will inhale as you lower your leg and exhale as you come up. Go for 2 to 3 sets of 15 to 20 reps.

Mia's Move for the Legs: The Leg Press (Two- and One-Legged Versions)

THE MOVE

Many people want more shape and strength in their legs but can't do squats (or don't want to). Not a problem! Leg presses are an excellent alternative. Unless you have a leg press machine in your home (lucky you!), then the gym will be the best place to find one.

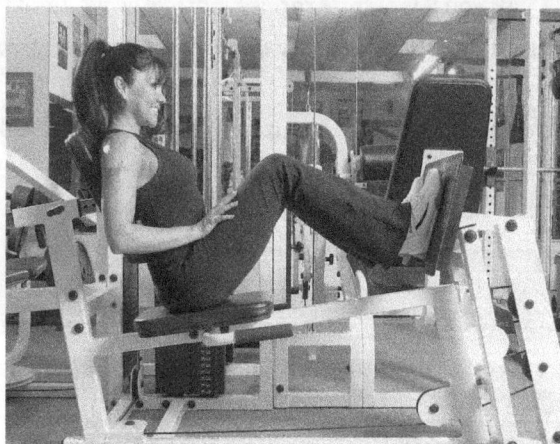

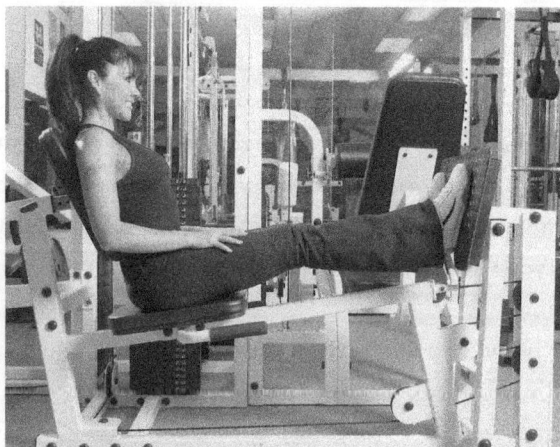

The leg press (and its many varieties) is the one where you're sitting on the machine's seat with your glutes and upper body positioned securely against the seat pads. Your feet will be placed in front of you and resting against the foot pad.

You'll see a few varieties of the leg press machine, with the biggest differences being the angle of how the platform functions and where your body will be seated and positioned. Regardless of which machine you use, keep these tips in mind.

HOW TO DO IT

Almost every leg press machine has a seat where you position your glutes and upper body and a foot platform on which to place your feet. Simply changing your foot position will allow you to direct the exercise to different areas on your legs.

Before you begin leg presses, you'll

want your body to be securely positioned by having your glutes firmly in the seat, your upper body solidly against the back pad, and your neck and head up as you look forward. Keep your abs tight, and with each hand hold onto the leg press side handles on either side of your body or resting on your thighs. Now let's look at the different moves you can do on these machines.

You can do adductor presses to work on your inner thighs. To do these presses, keep your legs perpendicular to the foot platform and use a wide stance, turning your feet out 20 to 30 degrees. Lower the weight and bring your legs out to the sides of your body. Squeeze your inner-thigh muscles as you push the weight back up.

The wider the foot position, the more you'll feel the exercise working the inner thighs. Do these in much the same way you would do your favorite leg press, except keep your feet wide and your toes pointed outward and placed high on the foot platform.

You can do regular leg presses to hit your overall thighs by placing your feet about shoulder-width apart and pointing them forward. Other leg presses work more on the outer thighs if you simply place your legs and feet close together (try having them touch each other) and keep your feet pointing straight ahead of you.

When you do regular leg presses, experiment with your foot placement (always keep your knees in a straight line over the toes). I like using full-range reps, although other people prefer short-range reps (lowering the weight about 4 to 10 inches).

Quick tip: For an extra contraction, lock your knees and rock back on your heels as you push your legs to their full extension, allowing your toes to rise off the platform.

For one-legged leg presses, the movement will essentially be the same as the two-legged presses, only you'll use one leg at a time.

The important things to remember when doing the one-legged leg presses are to reduce the weight (you simply won't be able to use as much as you would with both legs), be sure your working leg's foot position is near the center of the foot platform to ensure stability and safety, and do slower continuous reps to make the working leg's muscles burn. For any leg press version, you will inhale as you bend your knees and lower the foot platform toward your upper body and exhale as you extend your legs and push the foot platform forward to full extension. Do 2 to 3 sets of 10 to 15 reps.

THE MOVE

This is a simple move that's great for the back leg muscles (the hamstrings). To get the feel of it, simply stand erect. While keeping your upper body stationary, curl your lower leg up behind you. The upper leg will not move; only the lower leg and foot will come up. Curl that leg up to the point where you feel a good muscle contraction and then lower the leg back down. If you did that, then you've got the basics of the move down pat.

If you have a home gym multi-station (such as a universal-type weight machine), you should be able to do leg curls either standing up or lying down, or perhaps both. Regardless of which method you choose, be sure to follow these pointers.

HOW TO DO IT

First, in both versions of the leg curl, you'll want to isolate the hamstrings. You do that by keeping your upper legs in a fixed position and allowing only the knees to bend and the lower leg to move as you curl the weight up and down.

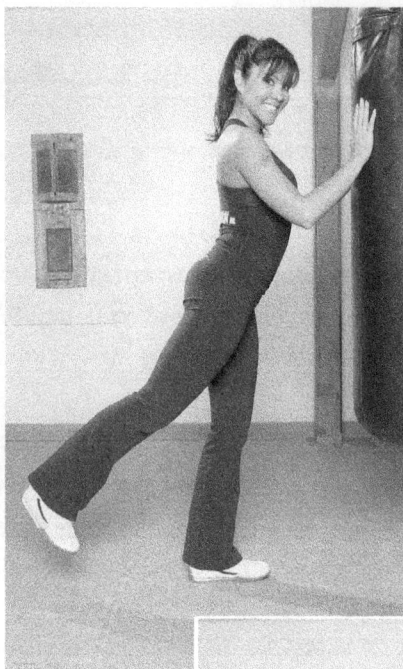

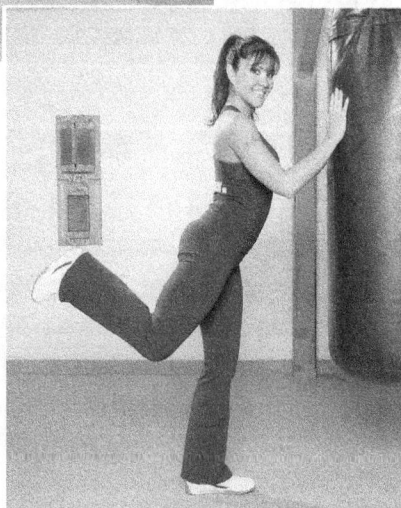

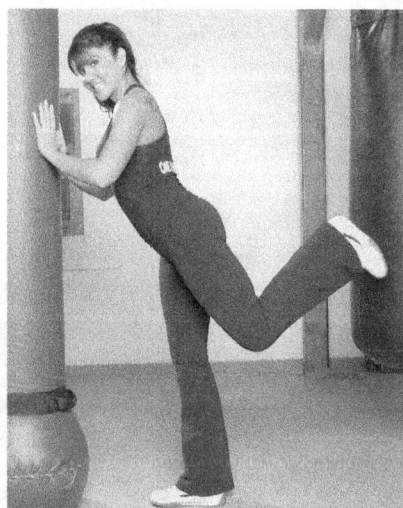

You'll also want to curl the weight up or back as far as you can and try to let the ankle pads touch your glutes. If you're able to bring them up this far, you can be sure that your hamstrings are getting a good stretch and contraction.

To do the lying leg curl, lie down on the leg curl bench and be sure your upper body and upper legs are firmly resting on top of the bench. Place your forearms on the bench underneath your chest, to elevate your upper body. Keep your neck and head down as you look forward. Position your lower legs so that the weight machine pad is just above your ankles at your lower calf area. Your toes will point down toward the floor. As you curl your lower legs up and back toward your glutes, try to drive your hips into the bench, which will help isolate the hamstrings, as well as protect your lower back.

For standing leg curls, keep your upper body erect with only a slight bend forward. Your neck and head will be erect as you look in front of you. Keep your abs tight. Focus on making the hamstring of the working leg the only muscle that moves as you do this exercise, and curl the back of the ankle pad up as high as you can until you feel the hamstring fully contract. Inhale before doing the exercise, exhale as you curl the leg up to a full contraction, and inhale as you lower the leg to the starting position.

Quick tip: For reps, I like to mix things up with this exercise. For example, in one workout, you might want to use a heavier weight and lower reps in the 6 to 10 range. In another workout, try doing 2 or 3 sets of 25 reps. For a third workout, do only one set of 50 to 100 reps. Mix it up all the time. Just aim to feel your leg muscles (hamstrings) squeeze, contract, and working hard.

Mia's Move for the Hamstrings: The Barbell/Dumbbell Dead Lift

THE MOVE

This is a truly great exercise for your hamstrings and lower back. Here, you have a choice. If you use a barbell, you'll stand erect, use a shoulder-width overhand grip, have a slight bend at the knees, and keep your head and neck erect as you look in front of you. Then bend your upper body forward over your feet and lower the barbell down to the level of your shins or the tops of your feet. (For more on how to figure out the right size of weights for you, see the list in the section titled "My Favorite Weight-Training Exercises" in this chapter.)

If you use dumbbells (as I do), you'll use the same body position as described above, only you'll bring the dumbbells down to the outsides of your calves and not directly in front of your shins, as with a barbell. More on this in a moment.

It's important to stretch really far down to get the most from this exercise, so if your range of motion isn't limited, you might want to stand on a wooden platform that's about 4 to 6 inches high so you can get even a greater stretch.

HOW TO DO IT

Let's do the dumbbell version. Begin the exercise by holding the dumbbells at your sides, with your arms straight down. Keep your upper body erect and your knees slightly bent. Keep your abs tight and your neck and head up as you look in front of you.

Now bend your upper torso forward with your head over your feet. As you lower your arms with the weights, rotate the dumbbells forward so they are in front of your shins and your palms are facing back toward your body. Be sure to keep the weights close to your legs.

DID YOU KNOW THAT... If you work in or visit the city, you can get a fabulous little workout that will shape and tone your lower legs and thin that hard-to-work ankle area simply by standing on the curb. While you wait for the light in order to cross the street, the trick is to place only your heels on the curb, while allowing your toes to touch the street pavement. Then you raise the fronts of your shoes up above curb level (or as high as possible) and do it for reps. Obviously, you need to be wearing sensible shoes and not stiletto heels to do this. These reverse toe raises are the secret to bringing out the best in your lower legs, and they will really help reduce your ankle size at the same time, thereby giving your legs a fantastic shape and appearance without your even going to the gym. Do this exercise each day, and watch what happens in just 10 days.

Also, keep your back slightly arched with your head up and in line with your upper back. You can keep your knees either locked or slightly bent, depending on how both of these positions feel. Bend far down enough so that your hamstrings are fully stretched, and then come back up to the starting position. Inhale as you lower your arms with the weights and exhale as you bring the weights back up to the starting position.

Quick tip: Some people can go down only to calf level. Others may stop a little higher, and some are flexible enough to hold the weights down below their feet (if they're using a platform). Do 6 to 8 reps per set and 2 to 3 sets.

Mia's Move for the Calves: The Calf Raise (Using Body Weight Only)

THE MOVE

Lucky for you, one of the best calf exercises can be done at home and without any machines, only by using the weight of your body and a few stair steps. Posture is key: your body is vertical, your neck and head are up and looking forward. Your abs are tight. Keep your knees locked or slightly bent, your toes are on a platform, and you simply go up and down, with only your ankles bending as your heels come up and down as high and low as they can.

Essentially, this is the same exercise you might do on a machine in a gym, but you'll do it a slightly different way. You will stand on a stair step and not on a machine, and you'll do lots of nonstop reps, but only one mega set of them.

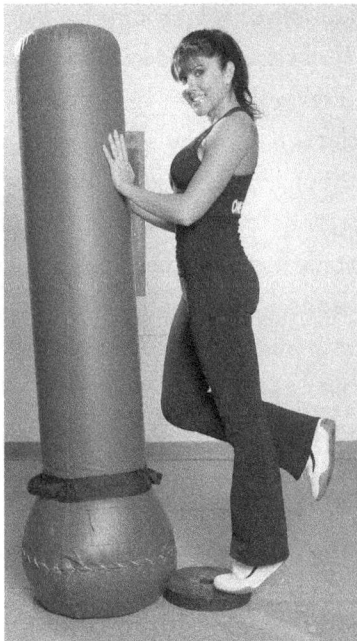

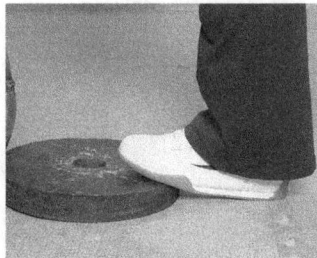

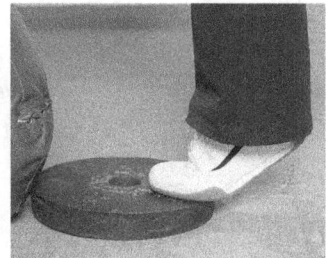

HOW TO DO IT

Calves respond incredibly well to either heavy weights or high reps—high, as in 50 reps and more. In fact, let's make it easy and forget counting reps. Just count minutes. Start off by doing two nonstop minutes of calf raises that go all the way up and all the way down.

Your body position will be similar to the way you'd stand on a machine to do a standing calf raise. Your body will be vertical, your neck and head up and looking straight ahead. Keep your abs tight. Place your hands on a column or the wall in front of you for balance, with your elbows bent and fingers pointing upward. Keep your knees locked or with a slight bend, your toes are on a platform, and you simply go up and down with only your ankles bending as your heels come up and down as high and low as they can. Inhale as you lower your heels to the bottom position, and exhale as you raise your heels up as far as you can for the peak contraction.

You'll feel your calves burn like never before, and you'll want to stop when it happens, but don't. This is the point where you make the exercise pay big rewards. When you can no longer do full-range reps, then do partial reps. Just keep your calves moving up and down until they can no longer do both.

I'll warn you, right here and now, that your calves will be sore for a good week or more if you perform these the way I just recommended. And the rule I want you to always remember is to never, ever work your calves again until they have completely recovered from your last calf workout. If you feel even the slightest degree of soreness, even if it's been a good week or more since the workout, then take another few days longer before you work them again. This may mean that you'll work your calves only three or four times a month and that's it. Oh, but wait until you see the results.

After a month or so of doing 2 nonstop minutes, increase the time to 3 minutes for the next month and then 4 minutes the following month after that.

Quick tip: Once you've increased the length of time, then start increasing the speed of your reps every once in a while for more intensity. Mix things up. And always remember to stretch the calves, by simply lowering your heels as far down as possible and holding them there for 20 to 40 seconds, after each calf workout.

THE MOVE

Okay, you've just perfected the standing calf raise by doing them with body weight only. Now it's time to do these on a machine. The important thing I want you to remember is the stretch at the bottom and the contraction at the top of the movement.

Your calves get worked every single day by walking. If you weigh 150 pounds, your calves get 150 pounds of resistance with each step, but they don't experience 150 pounds of resistance in the full range in which growth is stimulated.

HOW TO DO IT

Your body position will be similar to the way you did these on the body weight–only calf raise. Your body is vertical, your neck and head are up and looking straight ahead. Your abs are tight. Place your hands on the vertical bars of the machine for support. Keep your knees locked or with a slight bend, your toes are on a platform, and you simply go up and down with only your ankles bending as your heels come up and down as high and low as they can. Inhale as you lower your heels to the bottom position, and exhale as you raise your heels up as far as you can for the peak contraction.

Place the balls of your feet on the ends of the platform. Keep your body erect and move only your feet and ankles throughout the exercise. Pick a weight that is at least 50 percent heavier than your body weight, and do 2 to 3 sets with 10 to 12 reps per set.

Quick tip: Allow the weight to lower your heels all the way down to the floor below the platform in order to get a great stretch. Hold the weight in this position for 1 or 2 seconds, then rise up on your toes until your calves are fully contracted at the top position. Rest no longer than 30 seconds between sets.

For the Abdominals

Name one person who wouldn't like to have better-looking abs. Tough, isn't it? Abs not only look great, but they are such an important centerpiece of your body, affecting function, movement, flexibility, and strength. And you don't need razor-sharp six-pack abs to have a body that looks good, is healthy, and functions terrifically. Just watch what you eat (hint: go back to my nutrition tips for a shot of inspiration!), do these exercises, and you'll look great.

When it comes to the ab area and the various exercises you can do, here's the breakdown on which movements work on what areas: crunches typically hit the upper and middle abs; knee-ups work the lower abs; and trunk twists work the side abdominal region.

An important tip to remember when working the abs is to do non-stop reps and take only a minimal—not more than 25 seconds—rest between sets.

The other important factor is to do short-range movements. The abs can be worked with incredible intensity and effectiveness when constant tension is placed on them from doing nonstop, short-range reps. In many exercises, just a few inches of movement is all that it takes.

Mia's Move for the Abs: The Crunch

THE MOVE

This exercise is one of my favorites. It's simple, basic, and very effective if you pay attention to your body position and use nonstop reps. Crunches are similar to a sit-up in that the lower back and the glutes stay positioned on the floor or bench throughout the move, while the upper body lifts up and forward toward the legs as you contract the abs. There are a few more differences, which I'll describe.

HOW TO DO IT

Lie on the floor or on a flat bench. Bring your legs up with your knees bent and your legs together. Cross your arms in front of your upper body, or you can keep them at your sides. Your neck and head will be in line as you look up toward the ceiling.

Begin the exercise by raising your upper body off the ground and bringing it forward toward your knees. At the same time, bring your knees up and back toward your chin.

When your torso is in the up and fully contracted position, it should look similar to a U or V shape. Hold your body in this position for a count and squeeze the abs hard. Then slowly lower yourself back to the starting position. For the next rep in your set, try to bring your upper body farther forward as if you're trying to touch your knees with your upper body. On the third rep, don't raise your upper body so much or bring it so far forward, and instead bring your knees back farther as if you're trying to touch them to your chin.

Use this alternating pattern throughout your set; one rep of your knees back toward your face, the next rep of your upper body farther forward toward your knees. Back and forth, just like that. Inhale before the exercise, exhale as you bring your body up and forward, and inhale as you return your body to the starting position.

Quick tip: Throughout the exercise, don't allow your upper body to come back down and touch the floor or the bench. Keep it off the floor or the bench the whole time, since this will really make your abs work hard. Go for higher reps in the 30 to 50 range, and do 2 to 3 sets.

Mia's Move for the Abs: The Bicycle Crunch (with Legs Moving)

THE MOVE

This is quite similar to the regular crunch; however, as you move forward to crunch your upper torso, allow your knees to come back toward your chest at the same time and do small circular bicycle pedaling–type motions when your upper body is raised and closest to your knees. The body positioning, breathing, and execution will be the same as in the regular crunch.

HOW TO DO IT

For variation, you can do a straightforward crunch, a one side up/the other side up alternating type of crunch, or a combination of left side/straight forward/right side bicycle crunch.

As with all ab work, especially crunches, use nonstop short-range movements of only a few inches from start to finish, and keep the reps going without resting. This will make the abs burn and will work them very effectively.

Quick tip: Keep your upper body raised off the floor, and really bring your upper torso forward toward your knees as you pedal your legs. High reps in the 25 to 50 range work well on this. Go for 2 to 3 sets, and rest no longer than 15 to 20 seconds between sets.

Mia's Move for the Abs: The Knee-Up (Hanging or Lying)

THE MOVE

This is a terrific exercise for working your lower-abs and getting rid of the lower ab/waist area "paunch" that so many women want to make flatter and tighter. I'll show you two great ways to do these.

HOW TO DO IT

If you have a pull-up bar that will allow you to hang from it, go ahead and use it. The move is simple. Take an overhand grip about shoulder-width on the bar. Keep your arms straight and your body hanging down. Your neck and head will be up as you look forward. Keep your abs tight.

With your upper body erect and stationary, bring only your knees and legs up and back toward your stomach. Allow your upper body to bend or curve only slightly as you bring your knees up and back into your stomach area. Inhale before the exercise, exhale as you bring your legs up and back toward your stomach, and inhale as you return your legs back down to the starting position.

The second way to do these is simply by lying on the floor, a platform, or a flat

DID YOU KNOW THAT... If you want to move more gracefully and quickly and with more speed and power, a fun way to acquire this ability is by doing the fencing shuffle. And no, you won't need special clothes or a sword. The fencing shuffle mimics the moves of a fencer as he or she moves back and forth and from side to side. This is also a great way to strengthen your leg muscles and your connective tissue and will increase your agility and lateral stability. Begin by standing up straight, with a slight bend to the knees. Place your right or left foot forward (whichever feels most natural). Raise your heels to put more of your body weight on the balls of your feet. Move your body forward by using only the momentum of your body as you lean forward and spring off your toes. Your feet should come off the ground only a few inches as you move forward. Go straight ahead 6 to 12 inches and then spring back. Do the same thing to your left and right sides and then come back. Begin by moving only a few inches and then increase the distance you go forward or backward and from side to side as you get used to the movement.

bench. Put your hands, with your palms down, under your glutes so that your glutes are now elevated and off the floor, the platform, or the bench. Your neck and head will be erect as you look up. Keep your abs tight.

With both legs together, stretch your legs out in front of you. Be sure to raise your upper torso a few inches off the floor to keep tension on your abs.

Once your legs are fully extended in front of you, hold this for a count and then bend your knees and bring your legs up and back toward your upper body until your knees hit the ab area.

Quick tip: Again, it's crucial that you keep your feet and upper body raised off the floor from start to finish because this will keep constant tension on the lower abs. You will inhale before the exercise, exhale as your legs fully extend in front of you, then inhale as you bring your legs back up toward your upper body. Go for higher reps in the 25 to 50 range. Do 2 to 3 sets.

Mia's Move for the Abs: The Rocking Crunch

THE MOVE

This is another great variation on the crunch, but it's slightly more intense for even better results. The key is bringing the legs back and toward your upper body at the same time you're raising your upper body and bringing it forward toward your legs. As you'll see, the breathing and the body position are similar to what you've been doing, but with the following variations.

HOW TO DO IT

Lie on the floor or a flat bench with your legs up and your knees bent, while keeping your legs together. Raise your upper body and bring it forward toward your knees, while at the same time bringing your fully extended legs up and back toward your chin.

At the top position, your torso should be approaching the shape of a U or a V. On the next rep, don't bring your legs so far back but bring your upper body farther forward as if you're trying to touch your knees with your upper body.

On the third rep, don't raise your upper body so high or bring it so far forward and instead bring your legs and knees back farther as if you're trying to touch them to your chin. Inhale before the exercise, exhale as you raise your upper body and bring it forward and your legs back, and inhale as you return your upper and lower body to the starting position.

Quick tip: The rep cadence goes like this: the first rep is equal distance up for lower and upper body; on the second rep, your upper body is farther forward and your legs are lowered but not touching the floor; on the third rep, your upper body is lowered but not touching the floor and you bring your legs and knees farther back to try to touch your chin. Do 2 to 3 sets of 30 reps, with 10 reps each way.

Mia's Move for the Abs: The Standing Trunk Twist

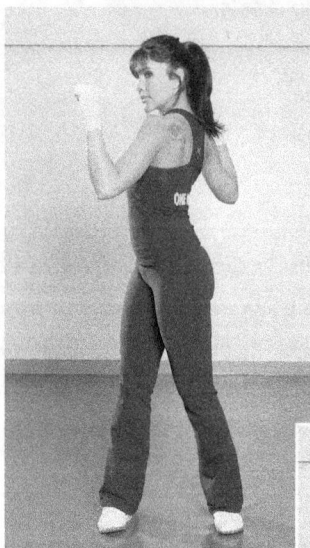

THE MOVE

These twists are great for working each side of your waist and trunk. The key to making these very effective is nonstop reps as you twist your upper body from side to side.

HOW TO DO IT

Stand erect with your feet about shoulder width apart. You can either lock your knees or bend them slightly if you prefer. Your upper body will be erect. Your neck and head are up as you look forward. Keep your abs tight.

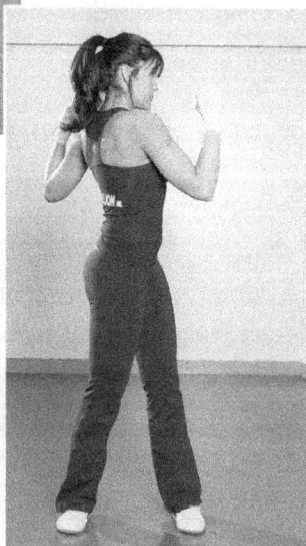

Use only your arms, with your fists up and close to your cheeks, or hold a broomstick while it rests on top of your shoulders behind your neck. Begin the move by doing the first twisting reps in a slower, more controlled range of motion to allow your body to warm up. Then, as your range of movement from left to right becomes easier and greater, twist your upper body just a little more with each rep, until you've comfortably reached your range-of-motion limits for each side.

During the move, allow your hips to freely move and swivel from side to side, but keep your lower body firmly positioned with your feet and knees facing forward. Inhale before the exercise, and exhale as you perform the move on each side, then inhale as you return your body to the center starting position.

Quick tip: Some people count reps (i.e., 25 reps for the right side, 25 reps for the left side) and others simply like to get in the zone and do continuous trunk twists for 1, 2, 3, or however many minutes nonstop.

Killer Cardio Strategies outside the Ring

You realize by now that if you want to develop a body that not only looks great but feels healthy, you need to do some type of aerobic training. Many people focus primarily on one type of cardio training and neglect the others. Yet to be balanced and to gain all of the benefits that will improve your health and appearance, you need to do equal amounts of training for the skeletal and the cardiovascular systems, as well as include a number of choices for your cardio workouts.

The great news is that it won't take you much time to get impressive results from both. You'll have more than enough ways to get your body in shape with the weights and my boxing workout, so don't even worry about that. Now, I'm going to tell you how to get your cardio act together, using equipment you've seen and are probably familiar with.

The Bike, the Stair Climber, and the Treadmill

The good old bike. You rode it as a kid, and there's no reason not to ride it as an adult. Whether you ride a stationary bike in your garage, bedroom, den, or living room or you want to ride a regular bicycle up and down the street, they are both excellent aerobic workouts.

The key thing to remember is to ride the bike long enough and fast enough to get your heart, blood, and lungs going. Lots of people sit on bikes and pedal aimlessly, expending little effort and never breaking a sweat. If you're content to go through the motions, that's fine, but if you want great results, you'll need to step up the pace.

With every type of aerobic training, shoot to train in your target heart range. To find this, simply take the number 220 and subtract your age in years (for example, if you're 35, it would be 220 − 35 = 185), then take that number (185, in our example) and keep your heart rate within 60 to 80 percent of it (that is, 185 × 60 percent = 111 beats per minute) while you train.

Whether you use a bike, a treadmill, or a stair stepper, try to do some type of aerobic training each day or every other day. Even if it's only for 10 or 12 minutes, at least it will get your heart, lungs, and body going.

You'd be surprised at how little aerobic training it takes to produce magnificent results. I know you've heard people say that unless you do 30 or more minutes of aerobic training at least three times a week, then you won't see much improvement.

Oh, yeah? I know many, many people who do between 12 and 25 minutes of aerobic activity per workout just three times a week and have gotten incredible results, simply because they knew how to train to maximize their efforts.

For the stair stepper, this means allowing only the balls of your feet to touch the steps, keeping your upper body erect and not bent forward as so many people do, and taking big, powerful strides up and down, instead of fast little chicken steps that move the steps up and down only a few inches.

For the treadmill, it means taking long strides, keeping your upper body erect, and swinging your arms vigorously. It also means walking at a brisk pace and, after a good warm-up (3 to 5 minutes), elevating the treadmill incline to 5 or more degrees and walking quickly on that incline for at least 10 minutes.

See, it's nothing complicated or fancy—simply good form and making your body work more intensely. Ahh, but I've saved the best for last.

The Power Walk

The coauthor of this book, Robert Wolff, had the honor of cowriting a book called *Building the Classic Physique—the Natural Way* with the late legendary Steve Reeves, the inventor of the modern Power Walk.

Steve Reeves was Mr. America and Mr. Universe, but he was probably more well known for his starring role in the movie *Hercules*. Reeves had the look, and he knew how to train for it in ways that made him a pioneer and are still emulated to this day.

Reeves developed a technique he called the Power Walk, and the only equipment you need to do it is a pair of shoes. The Power Walk can become your secret weapon. It will whip your body into great shape much faster than you imagined possible.

Steve Reeves told Robert that he believed long walks were a tonic to the ancient Greeks. "The best of all exercises," as Thomas Jefferson called it, has always been walking. Yet the Greeks, despite their wisdom, did not know the precise physical effects of walking. Now, even the American Medical Association's Committee on Exercise and Physical Fitness confirms that walking briskly, not merely strolling, is the simplest and also one of the best forms of exercise.

Reeves knew that ordinary walking can build heart and lung capacity only to a certain extent. Beyond that, the walker must go into something more strenuous. And Reeves realized that it's more difficult to walk fast than slow, more difficult to walk 3 miles than 1 mile, harder to walk on a 5 percent grade than on a level grade, and more difficult to walk with 15 additional pounds strapped to your body than with only your body weight.

He also said that the many benefits of his newly discovered method of walking became immediately apparent to him: he was breathing more deeply, his heart had picked up a few beats, and he wasn't sore the next day because the Power Walking had increased his circulation so much that it removed the lactic acid in his body.

To correctly do a Power Walk, you need to follow these guidelines:

- Length of stride—Keep it long and stretch your legs.
- Speed of movement—Vary the speed of Power Walking by using combinations of fast, medium, and slower walks.
- Distance traveled—Start off with short distances (i.e., less than a half-mile) and each week gradually go for longer distances.
- Degree of incline—Just like the treadmill in the gym, walking on an incline is harder (even at the same speed) than is walking the

same distance on a flat surface. Use a combination of flat and low-, medium-, and high-incline surfaces when you walk.

- Amount of weight carried—Once your Power Walks become easier and faster with your body weight, start adding wrist, ankle, or waist weights just above the hip bones as you walk (carry only a pound or two at first, because you can gradually add more later).
- Rhythmic breathing—Use rhythmic breathing by inhaling deeply for three strides (right, left, right) and then exhaling forcefully for three strides (left, right, left).
- When you Power Walk, there are four ways you can make it more intense and a better and more effective workout:

   Walk up hills.

   Carry additional weight as you walk.

   Walk longer distances.

   Walk faster.

When asked for his recommendations on how far someone needed to Power Walk to get in shape and stay in shape, Reeves said, "To get in shape, walk two to three miles. To stay in shape, walk one to two miles."

He also recommended keeping a log book to note your progress, because a log book can indicate how far you walked, how long it took you to walk it, descriptions about the road or the trail you walked (i.e., flat, inclines, declines, etc.), and whether you carried any extra weight when you walked.

As many people have known for a long time, walking (especially Power Walking) exercises the entire body and nearly all of your muscles—especially if you take long strides and swing your arms freely to the front and behind you as you walk.

Like Steve Reeves, for years I've recommended walking to people everywhere because it's one of the best exercises you can do, it has a very low risk of injury, anyone can do it, and you can do it whether you are young or old for the rest of your life. If you are not yet in the kind of condition you'd like to be in, walking, especially Power Walking, will get you there quickly. Although upper-body strength and the core muscles are important to your fitness success and conditioning, it's when you use the muscles below the abs—your legs—that you really start to burn calories and get into excellent cardio shape.

The good news is that when you walk, and especially when you Power Walk, you use your large lower-body muscles and smaller upper-body muscles at the same time, which will help you reach your goal that much quicker.

Steve Reeves told Robert about the following benefits of Power Walking for women:

> Power Walking is a great "bun burner" for women. When Power Walking, it is very important to use the heel-to-toe technique, but not in the traditional sense. The heel of the advancing foot should touch the ground with your knees slightly bent. As you roll to the flat foot position, straighten your leg and drive it forcefully to the rear with your buttocks muscles.
>
> It is extremely important to use the glutes as the driving force when pushing your leg to the rear. This is where the "bun-burning" effect, as I call it, comes from. As your front leg is driven back, the opposite leg should be thrust forward, taking as long a stride as possible. Always push with the buttocks and not the toes.
>
> To obtain maximum benefit from Power Walking, swing your arms back and forth in a pendulum-type of motion in opposition to your leg movement. Your arms should swing forward to an approximately 45-degree angle and back to approximately 30 degrees. Your left arm should swing forward as your right leg moves forward.
>
> Nothing can give you "instant fitness," but I can assure you that within one month of Power Walking three times a week for at least 15 minutes a session, you will see and feel dramatic results.

I agree! Start Power Walking and you'll see why.

Supercharging Your Workouts and Your Body—Even If You're Short on Time!

This is a fun section because Robert and I are going to give you some great new workouts that will produce amazing results. Use these tips and workouts to jump-start yourself when you lack motivation. They can help you get out of or avoid the inevitable ruts that many people experience when working out.

Look for something in each workout that can benefit you. Even if you don't have access to every piece of equipment that's used in a specific exercise, there may be something in the workout that you can try that will help you reach your goal.

Do as many or as few of these workouts as you like. There are no hard-and-fast rules. The most important thing is to have fun! Make working out something you look forward to, and you'll keep getting great results year after year after year.

Mia and Robert's Bootcamp Workout

This is a wonderful little workout that you can complete in less than twenty minutes and without going to the gym.

You can do up to three whole-body workouts in a five-day period; however, make sure you have at least one day of complete rest between workouts. After the third workout, take two complete days off from any training.

This workout is designed to accomplish a number of things:

- It gets you out of the gym. You can do this workout anywhere you'd like.

- It's a huge time saver because it has to be completed within twenty minutes.

- It works your body in fresh and different ways that you may not be accustomed to, because doing the same barbell, dumbbell and machine exercises can very quickly become boring.

- It combines the elements of body weight–only exercise (wherever possible) with endurance/resistance–type training that has a strong aerobic component.
- It gets you back to doing the kinds of exercise (away from the gym) you did when you were a kid and you had fun!

The key to making this workout benefit you is the near-zero rest factor between reps and exercises. I want you to put as much nonstop effort as you can into each rep, and then take *only* the least amount of rest you need to "catch your breath" before you get moving again. Here's the first movement.

Jump Rope (for 2 minutes)

If you have a jump rope, great. If you don't, get one. It'll be one of the best and cheapest investments you'll ever make. If you don't have or can't get a jump rope, then simply mimic the movement, doing everything you would do with the rope, but without actually holding the rope in your hands. You don't need to jump fast or high; just jump continuously for 2 minutes.

Breather (less than 1 minute)

After you've jumped for 2 nonstop minutes, you can take up to 60 seconds of rest, but *no* longer.

Standing High Front and Side Bent Leg Raises (for 2 minutes)

Think of these as if you're doing a martial arts kicking movement, similar to a Muay Thai kick, where you rotate your hip with each kick. The main things to remember are that you won't fully extend your legs and you'll do 10 nonstop reps for each leg before repeating the kicks with the opposite leg.

Begin by standing erect, bend your left knee, and raise your left leg directly out to the side of your body. Bring your leg no higher than hip level. Lower the

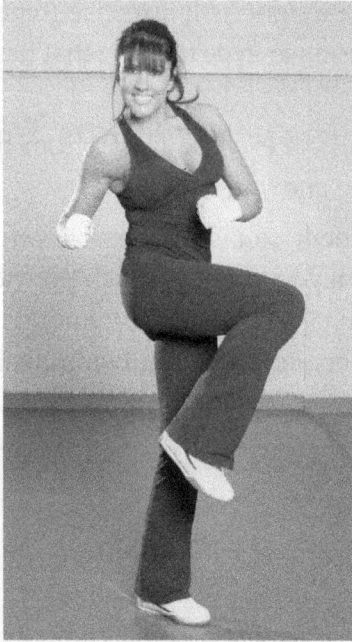

leg back down and then bring it back up again. Do not rest at either the top or the bottom of the movement. It should be a continuous motion of 10 nonstop reps. Then repeat this with the right leg.

In the second part of the exercise, do the same type of movement with your knee bent, but extend your leg straight out in front of your body. Again, do 10 nonstop reps with the left leg, then switch and do the same for the right leg.

On the third and final part of the exercise, go back to what you first did when you began the exercise for the left leg (the Standing Side Bent Leg Raise, then the Standing High Front Leg Raise), then do it the same way for the right leg. Go through a complete left/center/right/center leg movement sequence and then repeat the sequence. Do as many reps for the left side, the center, and the right side of your body as you possibly can for 2 minutes.

Breather (less than 1 minute)

After you've done 2 nonstop minutes, you can take up to 60 seconds of rest, but *no* longer.

Door Rows or Chins (for 2 minutes)

For your back and arms, my first choice would be for you to do chin-ups; however, I know these might present two problems:

1. You don't have a readily available chinning bar or access to one.
2. You may not be able to do very many reps even if you did. Not a problem. You can do some super-slow reps with door jamb/knob pulls.

Probably the easiest way to get used to the movement is by opening a door and placing the center of your body in line with the center of the outside part of the door (the side where the bolt and the latch are located). With both hands, grab hold of the door knobs, so that your left hand grabs the left knob and your right hand grabs the right knob. While holding the door, move your body back away from the door until your arms are fully extended and locked out. Don't worry that the door will move—it won't!

Now, bend down and lean back as far as you can, while keeping your arms straight. You'll find that positioning your feet forward and away from your upper body will give you more resistance. Keep your feet forward enough so that each foot is partway on one side of the door, to prevent it from moving.

Using only your arms and keeping your upper body stationary, you will now pull your body forward and toward the door. Once you get close to the door, lean back and *slowly* allow your upper body to return to the starting position.

The key to this is super-slow, focused, and concentrated nonstop reps, as you contract your back muscles when you reach the position *closest* to the door and stretch them as much as possible when you return to the starting position *farthest* from the door.

Breather (less than 1 minute)

After you've done 2 nonstop minutes, you can take up to 60 seconds of rest, but *no* longer.

Leg Elevated Push-ups (for 2 minutes)

We all know how to do a push-up. And if you are just starting out, it's much easier to do them with your knees bent on the floor, instead of with your knees raised off the floor as you balance on your toes.

But you're looking for the most effective way to do these because you have only two minutes. The trick is to elevate your feet so that they are *higher* than your upper body. That means you're going to have both legs and feet elevated and resting on a stationary platform or bench, and you will change your hand positions. So you will be doing these three different ways: with your hands placed out and far away from your body, with your hands placed midway between the farthest point away from your body and the closest point to your body, and with your hands placed directly under your body, under either the chest or the upper abs.

This is a tough one, so start off using the hand position that's most comfortable for you. Then start to experiment by moving your hands farther outward, farther inward, and even farther in front of you and see how each position feels and where it works your muscles.

Do as many reps as possible and rest only a few seconds, then do a few more reps. Keep up this "do-some-reps-then-rest-then-do-a-few-more-reps-then-rest" routine until you've done 2 minutes' worth of exercise.

For even more intensity, remember that the higher you raise your legs and feet above your upper body, the more difficult this exercise will be.

Breather (less than 1 minute)

After you've done 2 nonstop minutes, you can take up to 60 seconds of rest, but *no* longer.

Continuous Dumbbell Side Laterals Supersetted to Bent-Over Dumbbell Simultaneous Curls (for 2 minutes) (see page 72)

This is the only superset (i.e., doing two back-to-back sets of different exercises with the absolute minimum amount of rest between the sets) in the workout and one you'll like a lot. You'll need two dumbbells.

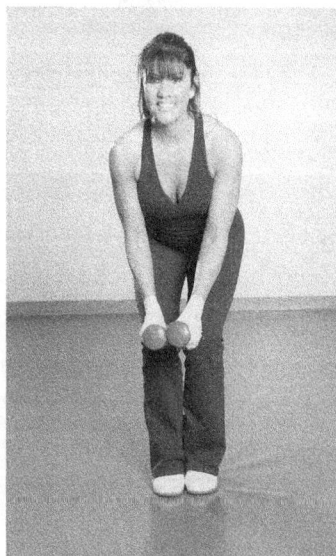

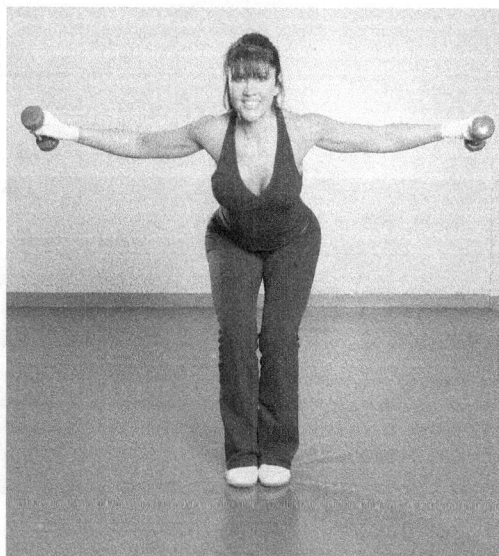

You'll begin by doing a set of nonstop standing dumbbell side laterals. Do some of the reps by lifting the weights straight out to your sides (in a direct line with your upper body), other reps with your arms slightly in front of you as you raise the dumbbells, and another group of reps with your arms directly in front of your body. Do 1 minute of continuous nonstop reps, and *don't* do these slowly. Pick up the pace and really keep the weights moving quickly. Do *not* let your arms rest at either the top or the bottom position of the exercise. Keep them moving!

After you've done 1 nonstop minute of dumbbell laterals, bend your upper body forward and bring both arms in front so that they're hanging straight down under you. Now bring your arms slightly forward (so that they are at an angle and not at 90 degrees) and begin to curl both dumbbells up at the same time. At the top of the movement, really squeeze and contract your biceps and turn the dumbbells outward (supinate) so that the little fingers on both hands are higher than the thumbs. Then lower the dumbbells *all* the way down until your arms are fully extended, do it again, and keep doing it like this for 1 minute.

As soon as you've done 1 minute of the dumbbell curls, stand up straight again and do your last minute of side laterals, immediately followed by your last minute of dumbbell curls, and that's it!

Breather (less than 1 minute)

After you've done 3 nonstop minutes, you can take up to 60 seconds of rest, but *no* longer.

Stretch and Cool-Down

Now go through your favorite stretching movements (which you'd do either before, during, or after your workout), and be sure that you stretch all of the body parts you worked. (See pages 55, 61, 65, and 70 for stretching exercise instructions.) Just do some nice and easy "stretch and relax" movements for 10 seconds or so for each body part and, my friend, you have accomplished something new and different to add to your toolbox of workouts and exercises.

The Thirty-Day Jump-Start

Are you looking for a sure cure for the "I'm in a rut" blues? It's called the 30-Day Jump-Start, and it can transform your body.

Because your body quickly habituates (translation: gets used to doing the same thing), oftentimes you'll need to not only do something completely different, but do it in unconventional ways. If you've been working out using the same kinds of exercises, with the same weights and reps, then your body could benefit from something completely different.

Try doing 50 percent less sets and 50 percent less exercises, but double your workout intensity. That is, spend less time working out, but lift heavier weights (only after a good warm-up) during the workout.

When I say "heavier," I'm not talking about an extra 5 or 10 pounds. I mean using near-maximum-ability weights for less reps, say 3 to 6 reps instead of 10 to 12. Be prepared to feel a bit sore after each workout, but the soreness will quickly go away as your body breaks out of its rut. You'll become stronger and firmer in areas you may have thought could not change.

The key is to use this training and any other type you'd like to try for the next 30 days, and then you can go back to a maintenance program, the kind that you were on before you began the 30-Day Jump-Start. You may find that doing the 30-Day Jump-Start every four months is just the ticket to maximize your progress for years to come.

The Anywhere, Anytime Workout

Here's something you can do anywhere, anytime, and it will give you a potent little "mini-workout" without your going to the gym or touching a weight. It's called "tense and relax," and it works like this: Pick any muscle, let's say the biceps. Flex that arm until you feel the biceps contracting and tensing. Hold the biceps in that tensed position for anywhere from 4 to 10 seconds. Really tense it as hard as you can for the entire 4 to 10 seconds. Let that arm relax, and do the same thing for the other arm.

For the chest, put both arms straight out in front of you and don't allow them to touch as you squeeze your chest together. For the triceps, simply let an arm hang down to your side and tense the triceps as you straighten the arm.

The trick is to keep the maximum amount of tension for 4 to 10 seconds on the muscle you want to work. The harder the contraction, the better the result.

The Holistic Training Principle Workout

Your muscle cells contain proteins and energy systems that respond differently to various levels of exercise. Muscle-fiber proteins get larger when they perform against high-resistance loads. The cells' aerobic systems (mitochondria) respond to high-endurance training. That's why it's important for your training to include a variety of heavy weights/low reps to light weights/high reps in order to maximize your results.

This principle means that you will always use a combination of training techniques within every workout you do. For example, you may come to the gym with a plan that today will be your heavy weights/lower reps workout day, only to discover when you try this that despite your best efforts and using the heavy weights and the low reps, nothing is happening. Your body isn't responding well to that kind of training.

So, what to do? Two things—perhaps a "jump-start" of a few sets of light weights and high pumping reps is all that's necessary to get your body ready for that heavy weights/low reps workout. Or maybe you need to devise a complete change of plans right there on the spot. That is, flip your training around and make that week a light weights/blood pumping/muscle flushing workout week, then take a nice 2 or 3 full days of rest and watch what happens when you come back the following week and hit it hard and heavy.

The point to remember is that your body is not a machine that will respond exactly how you think it should, whenever you want it to. It's a beautiful complex system of emotions, muscle, bone, tissue, blood, and so many other synergistic parts. You will always know, from the start of the first rep of your workout to the last rep, how it's responding to today's workout.

So stay flexible, adaptable, and open to changing how you train, from that first rep to the last set. Set nothing in stone regarding what you should do today and how you should do it. Listen to your body. It'll tell you exactly how it wants to be trained today. That's holistic training, and that's what I call smart.

The Six Weeks On and One Week Off Workout

This will be a fun way for you to train and will produce great results if you follow a simple premise: for every six weeks of training, take one complete week off.

Many people have found that this workout contains just the right amount of training and has the key elements of training cycling: increased conditioning and endurance, power peaking, and progressively rising strength that is timed to peak on week 6. And its reward, after the last workout on week 6, is a much-needed and much-welcomed one full week off.

The key components of this workout are:

- It has 6 weeks of training, followed by 1 full week off.

- On week 1, you train at 60 percent of your maximum capacity.

- On week 2, you train at 70 percent of your maximum capacity.
- On week 3, you train at 80 percent of your maximum capacity.
- On week 4, you train at 90 percent of your maximum capacity.
- On week 5, you train at 80 percent of your maximum capacity.
- On week 6, you train at 100 percent of your maximum capacity.

When I talk about "maximum capacity," for this workout, that means your 3-rep maximum best.

For example, if the most you can do on the bench press is 150 pounds for 3 reps, then this would be your 100 percent maximum capacity.

You simply take 60 percent of that 150 pounds (90 pounds) and that's what you'd use for week 1. For week 2, you'd use 105 pounds. On week 3, you'd use 120 pounds, and so on.

Take some time before you begin your workout to figure out which exercises you'll want to use and what your 60 percent through 100 percent numbers are for each exercise.

Exercises, Sets, and Reps

For each of your body parts, make a list of the exercises your body responds best to. For example, for the chest, the most effective exercises you may have found are dumbbell inclines or dumbbell flys (perhaps pec dec or cable cross-overs if you have access to a gym). That would be the group of chest exercises you'd pick from during the six-week period when you work your chest. Now, make a list like that for every one of your body parts.

For sets and reps, use these ranges:

- For week 1, 60 percent training, do 2 to 3 exercises per body part and 12 reps per exercise.
- For week 2, 70 percent training, do 2 to 3 exercises per body part and 10 reps per exercise.
- For week 3, 80 percent training, do 2 to 3 exercises per body part and 8 reps per exercise.
- For week 4, 90 percent training, do 2 to 3 exercises per body part and 5 reps per exercise.

- For week 5, 80 percent training, do 2 exercises per body part and 7 reps per exercise.
- For week 6, 100 percent training, do 1 exercise per body part and 1 to 3 reps for that exercise.

Note: During this 6-week workout, keep your cardio training to no more than 20 minutes per workout and at no higher than a fat-burning intensity level, and do your cardio work *after* the weight workout.

The Four-Zone Workout

Whether we like it or not, society too often defines us by our body parts. Women seem to want certain body parts to look especially sexy, while guys want other parts to be buff. Add this to the fact that society's favorite body part of the month changes so fast, and it makes your head spin.

Just look at how quickly magazine covers and articles change their priorities each month. We have infomercials telling us that abs are the magic muscle to make us look and feel good. Then, only a few months later, the message is, Forget the abs, it's now legs. Who can keep up? Who wants to?

I'm a big believer in finding balance in our lives, and this is especially true when it comes to working out and building and toning our bodies. Still, women are going to want certain body parts to look better than others. And on many lists and polls that ask people what they would like to change about how they look, certain body parts are often found at the top for women.

To help you achieve the look you want, Robert and I have created a great specialized workout for women that focuses specifically on the top-of-the-list body parts and includes some of the best exercises and workouts we've seen to transform those body parts.

Flat Stomach Area (Front Core)

Do one or two of the following ab exercises each workout, and make sure that for each workout you do different exercises than you used for the previous workout. Don't rest between reps, and don't allow the abs to relax. The only rest the abs should get are the 15- to 20-second breathers between sets and when you move to the next ab exercise. Think constant tension and short range of movement, and your abs will respond beautifully!

The Rocking Crunch

THE MOVE

This is another great variation on the crunch but is slightly more intense for even better results. As you'll see, the breathing and the body position are similar to what you've been doing, but with the following variations.

HOW TO DO IT

Lie on the floor or a flat bench with your legs up and your knees bent and legs together. Raise your upper body and bring it forward toward your knees, while at the same time you bring your fully extended legs up and back toward your chin.

At the top position, your body should be approaching the shape of a U or a V. On the next rep, don't bring your legs so far back but bring your upper body farther forward, as if you're trying to touch your knees with your upper body.

On the third rep, don't bring your upper body so far up and forward and instead bring your legs and knees back farther as if you're trying to touch them to your chin. Inhale before the exercise, exhale as you raise your upper body and bring it forward and your legs back, and inhale as you return your upper and lower body to the starting position.

Quick tip: The rep cadence goes like this: the first rep is equal distance up for the lower and the upper body; on the second rep, the upper body comes farther forward and the legs are lowered but not touching the floor; on the third rep, the upper body is lowered but not touching the floor and the legs and the knees come back to try to touch the chin. Do 2 to 3 sets of 30 reps, 10 reps each way.

The Bicycle Crunch (with Legs Moving)

THE MOVE

This is quite similar to the regular crunch; however, as you come forward to crunch your upper torso, allow your knees to come back toward your chest at the same time and do small circular bicycle pedaling–type motions when your upper body is raised and closest to your knees. The body positioning, the breathing, and the execution will be the same as in the regular crunch.

HOW TO DO IT

For variation, you can do a straightforward crunch, a one side up/the other side up alternating type of crunch, or a combination of left side/straight forward/right side bicycle crunch.

As with all ab work, especially crunches, use nonstop short-range movements of only a few inches from start to finish, and keep the reps going without resting. This will make the abs burn and will work them very effectively.

Quick tip: Keep your upper body raised off the floor and really bring your upper body forward and toward your knees as you pedal your legs. High reps in the 25 to 50 range work well for this. Go for 2 to 3 sets and rest no longer than 15 to 20 seconds between sets.

The Knee-Up (Hanging or Lying)

THE MOVE

This is a terrific exercise for working your lower abs and getting rid of the lower ab/waist area "paunch" that so many women want to make flatter and tighter. I'll show you two great ways to do knee-ups.

HOW TO DO IT

If you have a pull-up bar that will allow you to hang from it, go ahead and use it. The move is simple. Take an overhand grip, with your hands about shoulder width apart on the bar. Keep your arms straight and your body hanging down. Your neck and head will be up as you look forward. Your abs will be tight.

While keeping your upper body erect and stationary, bring your knees up and back toward your stomach. You legs will bend as you bring the knees up.

Allow your upper body to bend or curve only slightly as your knees come up and back into your stomach area. Inhale before the exercise, exhale as you bring your legs up and back toward your stomach, and inhale as you return your legs back down to the starting position.

The second way you can do these is simply by lying on the floor, a platform, or a flat bench. Put your hands, with your palms down, under your glutes so that your glutes are now elevated and off the floor, the platform, or the bench. Your neck and head will be erect as you look up. Your abs will be tight.

While keeping both legs together, extend them out in front of you. Be sure to keep your upper torso raised a few inches off the floor to keep tension on the abs. Once your legs are fully extended in front of you, hold this for a count and then bend your knees and bring your legs up and back toward your upper body until your knees hit the ab area.

Quick tip: Again, it's essential that you keep your feet and upper body raised off the floor from start to finish, as this will put constant tension on the lower abs. You will inhale before the exercise, exhale as your legs fully extend in front of you, then inhale as you bring your legs back up toward your upper body. Go for higher reps in the 25 to 50 range. Do 2 to 3 sets.

The Standing Trunk Twist

THE MOVE

These are great for working each side of your waist and trunk. The key to making these very effective is nonstop reps as you twist your upper body from side to side.

HOW TO DO IT

Stand erect with your feet about shoulder-width apart. You can either lock your knees or bend them slightly if you prefer. Your neck and head are up as you look forward. Keep your abs tight.

With your arms up and close to your shoulders and your fists facing your cheeks, or holding a broomstick with hands shoulder width apart as the broomstick rests on top of your shoulders behind your neck, begin the move by doing the first twisting reps with a slower, more controlled range of motion to allow your body to warm up. Then, as your range of movement from left to right becomes easier and greater, twist your upper body a little more with each rep, until you've comfortably reached your range-of-motion limits for each side.

During the move, allow your hips to freely move and swivel from side to side, but keep your lower body firmly positioned with your feet and knees facing forward. Inhale before the exercise, and exhale as you perform the move on either side, then inhale as you return your body to the center starting position.

Quick tip: Some people count reps (i.e., 25 reps for the right side/25 reps for the left side), and others simply like to get in the zone and do continuous trunk twists for 1, 2, 3, or however many minutes nonstop.

Tight, Round Glutes

You'll find numerous exercises and machines that will work the glutes, but many people have gotten great results from doing a select few exercises. Here they are.

The Squat (see "The Squat" on page 125)

THE MOVE
One of the best exercises you can do for your legs is the squat. This exercise not only targets the muscles on the front of the legs (the quads), but also works the hamstrings, the glutes, and the lower back at the same time. Proper form is essential when performing the squat. Keep your upper body erect, with your head up as you look forward, and let your upper leg stop about parallel to the floor when you reach the bottom of the movement. Be sure to keep your knees in line with your toes and do not let your knees go forward over the toes at the bottom position. Squats can be tough, but they are a great leg exercise, indeed!

HOW TO DO IT
Stand erect, with your head up as you look forward, and place your feet about shoulder width apart, pointing in front of you. Keep your abdominals pulled in. Bring your arms out and in front of your body. Cross your arms so that your hands are resting on opposite elbows. Inhale, and while keeping

your arms out in front of you, shift your weight back onto your heels and bend your knees to squat down. (Pretend there's a chair behind you and you're about to sit in it as you lower yourself into a squatting position.) Go no lower than having your upper legs parallel to the floor. Stopping a little higher than parallel is just fine.

As you get ready to return to the top starting position, exhale and squeeze your glutes and bring your body up. Inhale at the top position. Keep your chest lifted from start to finish, and don't sit lower than the upper-legs-parallel-to-the-floor point or let your knees go forward past your toes. Go for 2 to 3 sets of 12 to 15 reps.

If you're doing back squats with a barbell and weights, let the bar rest high on your upper back/shoulder area somewhere on the traps. Take a grip on each side of the bar that's slightly wider than your shoulders. Place your feet about shoulder-width apart and turn them slightly out. For more stability, you may want to slightly elevate your heels an inch or two. Using two weight plates works great as a heel raise.

Use the same exercise form as just described, but arch your lower back slightly and keep your head up as you look straight ahead. Squat down until your thighs are about parallel to the floor. Always make sure your knees travel in a direct line over your big toes.

You will inhale before you squat, as you bend your knees and lower the weight to the bottom position, and exhale as you bring your body and the weight up to the starting position. Do 2 to 3 sets of 8 to 12 reps.

Quick tip: For variety and to work the inner thighs, try doing wide-stance squats. Essentially, you'll do them the same way you did the regular squat, using

<table>
<tr><td>DID
YOU
KNOW
THAT...</td><td>Almost everyone loves chocolate but doesn't love the high calories it contains. And with more news coming out about the health benefits of eating "moderate" amounts of chocolate every so often, is there a way you can have that chocolate and feel good about it, too? You bet. Whenever possible, try using unsweetened cocoa powder in your recipes because cocoa powder is chocolate, but with most of the fat removed.</td></tr>
</table>

the same upper-body positioning. The only difference is the placement of your feet. Keep your legs and feet about 2 to 3 feet apart and turn the feet outward (always making sure that your knees are in line with the big toes, but do not go forward over the toes), to allow the exercise to work your inner thighs. Higher reps in the 12 to 16 range work well. Do 2 to 3 sets.

The Lunge and the Walking Lunge (see "The Walking Lunge" on page 126)

THE MOVE

I'm sure you've seen people do lunges, but many do them incorrectly despite using the right form, because they do them with so little intensity that the lunges produce no noticeable results.

The trick is to use great form but make your quads burn by doing nonstop reps. That means no resting at the top of the exercise for a second or two and then going down again. I want you doing nonstop reps, and do all the reps for the set for each leg before you change legs.

Be sure to keep your knee in a direct line over your big toe during the exercise to prevent injury. I suggest going down enough that your upper leg is lower than parallel to the floor. I think you'll feel the exercise more.

Always keep the quad of your nonworking leg in a direct line with your upper torso and not in front or behind. You can either hold the dumbbells down at your sides or up next to your shoulders, as if you are doing a press. Keep your palms facing your cheeks.

HOW TO DO IT

The walking lunge is one of my favorite exercises to target not only the fronts and the backs of the legs, but the glutes as well. I see many women doing lunges, but very few do them correctly. Or perhaps I should say, "effectively." As with any exercise, it's easy to just go through the motions, but that's not what you want to do. You want results, and you'll get them by focusing directly on the muscles and using great form. The good news is, you don't even need to use weights (your body weight alone will do!) to get terrific results.

Begin by standing up straight with your legs and feet together. Keep your chest raised, your upper body erect, your back straight, and your abdominals pulled in, while your head looks forward. With your right foot, take a large step forward. Now drop your left knee down toward the ground, and try to keep it directly under your body and in as close a direct line with your upper body as you can. Be sure to keep your upper body upright and facing forward while you're at the bottom position.

Now bring your upper body up and move your left leg forward and bring your right leg down, directly under your body, with the right knee touching the floor, and repeat the same exercise sequence.

Quick tip: Keep moving forward (one leg, then the other) until you reach the end of the room or someplace where you can turn around and repeat the lunges for your next set. You will inhale as you lower your leg and exhale as you come up. Go for 2 to 3 sets of 15 to 20 reps.

Inner Thighs

The Leg Press with Feet Wide (Two- and One-Legged Versions)

THE MOVE

Many people want more shape and strength in their legs but can't do (or don't want to do) squats. Not a problem! Leg presses are an excellent alternative.

Unless you have a leg press machine in your home, then the gym will be the best place to find one. You'll see a few varieties, with the biggest differences being the angle of how the platform functions and where your body will be seated and positioned. Regardless of which machine you use, keep these tips in mind.

HOW TO DO IT

Almost every leg press has a seat where you position your glutes and upper body and a foot platform on which to place your feet. Simply changing your foot position will allow you to direct the exercise to different areas on your legs.

Before you begin leg presses, you'll want your body to be securely positioned by having your glutes firmly in the seat, your upper body solidly against the back pad, and your neck and head up as you look forward. Keep your abs tight, and with each hand hold onto the leg press handles on either side of your body or keep your hands on your thighs. Now let's look at the different moves you can do on these machines.

You can do adductor presses to work on your inner thighs. To do these presses, keep your legs perpendicular to the foot platform and use a wide stance, turning your feet out 20 to 30 degrees. Lower the weight and bring your legs out to the sides of your body. Squeeze your inner-thigh muscles as you push the weight back up.

The wider the foot position, the more you'll feel the exercise working the inner thighs. Do these in much the same way you would do your favorite leg press, except keep your feet wide and your toes pointed outward and placed high on the foot platform.

You can do regular leg presses to hit your overall thighs by placing your feet about shoulder-width apart and pointing them forward. Other leg presses work more on the outer thighs if you simply place your legs and feet close together (try having them touch each other) and keep your feet pointing straight ahead of you.

When you do regular leg presses, experiment with your foot placement (always keep your knees in a straight line over the toes). I like using full-range reps, although other people prefer short-range reps (lowering the weight about 4 to 10 inches).

Quick tip: For an extra contraction, lock your knees and rock back on your heels as you push your legs to their full extension, allowing your toes to rise off the platform.

For one-legged leg presses, the movement will essentially be the same as the two-legged presses, only you'll use one leg at a time.

The important things to remember when doing the one-legged leg presses are to reduce the weight (you simply won't be able to use as much as you would with both legs), be sure your working leg's foot position is near the center of the foot platform to ensure stability and safety, and do slower continuous reps to make the working leg's muscles burn. For any leg press version, you will inhale as you bend your knees and lower the foot platform toward your upper body and exhale as you extend your legs and push the foot platform forward to full extension. Do 2 to 3 sets of 10 to 15 reps.

Outer Thighs

Squats (Legs Together)

Here's a little trick to remember whenever you work your legs. By simply changing your foot position, you change where the exercise will hit the muscle. Having your feet in a wide stance hits your inner thighs; having your feet together works your outer thighs. So, where do you think squats with your feet together will hit? That's right, your outer thighs. Here are a few other helpful tips.

The Squat (see "The Squat" on page 125)

THE MOVE

One of the best exercises you can do for your legs is the squat. This exercise not only targets the front leg muscles (the quads), but also works the hamstrings, the glutes, and the lower back at the same time. Proper form is essential when performing the squat. You want your upper body to be upright, your head up as you look forward, and your upper leg stopping about parallel to the floor when you reach the bottom of the movement. Be sure to keep your knees in line with your toes, and do not let your knees go forward past the toes at the bottom position. Squats can be tough, but they are a great leg exercise, indeed!

HOW TO DO IT

Stand erect, with your head up as you look forward, and place your feet about shoulder width apart, pointing in front of you. Keep your abdominals pulled in. Bring your arms out and in front of your body. Cross your arms so that your hands are resting on opposite elbows. Inhale, and while keeping your arms out in front of you, shift your weight back onto your heels as you bend your knees to squat down. (Pretend there's a chair behind you and you're about to sit in it as you lower yourself into a squatting position.) Go no lower than having your upper legs parallel to the floor. Stopping a little higher than parallel is just fine.

As you get ready to return to the top starting position, exhale and squeeze your glutes and bring your body up. Inhale at the top position. Keep your chest lifted from start to finish, and don't sit lower than the upper-legs-parallel-to-the-floor point or let your knees go forward past your toes. Go for 2 to 3 sets of 12 to 15 reps.

If you're doing back squats with a barbell and weights, let the bar rest high on your upper-back/shoulder area somewhere on the traps. Take a grip on each side of the bar that's slightly wider than your shoulders. Place your feet about shoulder-width apart and turn them slightly out. For more stability, you may want to slightly elevate your heels an inch or two. Using two weight plates works great as a heel raise.

Use the same exercise form that was just described, but add a slight arch to your lower back and keep your head up and looking straight ahead. Squat down until your thighs are about parallel to the floor. Always make sure your knees travel in a direct line over your big toes.

You will inhale before you squat and exhale as you bring your body and the weight up to the starting position.

Use nonstop near-lock-out reps. The trick is to keep your legs constantly burning. You do this by stopping each rep about three-quarters of the way at the top, then going back down again for the next rep. Do 3 to 4 sets of 15 to 20 nonstop three-quarter reps.

Quick tip: For variety and to work the inner thighs, try doing wide-stance squats. Essentially, you'll do them the same way you just did the regular squat, using the same upper-body positioning. The only difference is the placement of your feet. To work your inner thighs, you'll keep your legs and feet about 2 to 3 feet apart and turn your feet outward (always making sure that your knees align with the big toes, but don't go forward past the toes). Higher reps in the 12 to 16 range work well. Do 2 to 3 sets.

Leg Press (Feet Together)

Here you go again, this time with your feet together to hit your outer thighs.

Do one set with your feet high on the platform, one set with your feet positioned in the middle of the platform, and one set with your feet low on the platform. How did you feel during each set? Where did you feel it?

Change your seat position, too. For one set, have the seat all the way declined. For another set, raise the seat a few notches. Keep your feet in the same position when you move the seat.

You'll want to figure out whether you feel any differences when you adjust your body position by moving the seat. Once you've determined that, then change your foot position on the platform, and use the combinations where you feel effects of the exercise the most.

Do 3 to 4 sets of 18 to 22 nonstop three-quarter reps.

Standing Side Leg Raise (Knee Bent and Body Weight Only)

To do these leg raises, forget about securing a strap attached to a low pulley around your ankles. Simply use your body weight, and it'll work great.

Stand erect and with your right hand hold a vertical bar on a machine or the back of a chair for balance. Raise your left leg up and directly out to your left side. Bend your knee so that your calf and your foot face behind your body.

While keeping your upper body erect, raise your left leg up as far as possible. Aim for waist level, if you can. If you're really limber, try to go a bit higher, but keep your upper body upright throughout the exercise. Keep your knee bent and behind you as you lower and raise your leg, and don't let it touch the floor until you've done 20 reps.

Do 3 to 4 sets of 20 nonstop reps per side.

Shapely Shoulders

Standing or Seated Dumbbell Lateral Raise
(Side, Front, and Bent-Over) (see page 136)

You don't need to lift heavy weights to develop strong, shapely shoulders. And put away those shoulder pads that you've tucked inside your tops. You'll soon not need them. The shoulders respond especially well to nonstop reps and to reps.

Since the shoulders (deltoids) comprise three separate muscles (front, side, and rear), by simply changing your upper-body position, you can work all three with the same exercise.

Begin with front raises and do one arm at a time. Keep your upper body erect, and, with your arm fully extended, raise the dumbbell up and directly out in front of you until it comes to shoulder level, with your palm facing down. Hold it there for 1 to 2 seconds, then slowly lower it and do the same for the other side. Do 8 to 10 reps.

After the last rep, bring the dumbbells down to your sides, then raise both arms up and directly out to your sides so that your arms holding the weights are in a straight line with your upper body, with your palms facing down. You can slightly bend your elbows, but not much. Do 8 to 10 reps.

After the last rep, lower the weights down and bend your upper body forward. If you're seated, your upper body will be over your legs. If you're standing, your upper body will be bent over at about 80 to 90 degrees from the floor. Extend your arms with the weights up and out to your sides, just as you did in the last exercise of side laterals, with your palms facing down. Do 8 to 10 reps. Do 2 to 3 sets of these three nonstop delt exercises.

Mia's Quick Tips for Dropping the Pounds

Looking and feeling great is something I want you to experience for the rest of your life. Anything worth having (like a body that looks and feels fabulous and healthy) is worth taking the time to achieve it, so I want you to avoid the desire for (and the disappointment of) a "quick fix."

I know there may be times in your life when special events come up and you would really a like a jump-start on losing a few pounds and slimming down faster, so I'll give you some tips that have worked well for me.

However, remember that these are only to be used *occasionally* and when you absolutely need them.

- Lifting weights is great for toning, but it takes months for you to see the results. Jump-start your weight-loss routine with cardiovascular exercise to get your heart pumping. Excessive perspiration from running, speed walking, working out on aerobic gym equipment, and jumping rope will help you de-bloat and lose inches and pounds quickly. I recommend doing cardio several times a week as a warm-up for 10 to 15 minutes or as a workout for at least 30 minutes, to really get your heart rate going.

- Spice up your workouts by adding punches to your routine. Lunges and crunches are important for toning abs, thighs, and glutes. By adding punches to lower-body workouts, you'll also be working your arms and back, making for a full-body workout in less time. The added moves also keep your heart rate elevated, contributing to more perspiration and increased calories burned.

- Eliminate white carbohydrates while you eat lean protein for a couple of weeks to quickly drop a few pounds or jump-start your fitness program. Lean protein is important for growth and to build and repair bones and muscles. Fill your diet only with fibrous carbohydrates, such as berries, spinach, broccoli, cauliflower, and apples, as well as protein from poultry, fish, eggs, and low-fat dairy products. You'll also find it helpful for your fat-loss and conditioning goals if you cut back on alcoholic beverages and fried foods.

- Too much salt isn't healthy, especially for someone who is trying to drop a few pounds. Excess salt can result in high blood pressure, and it causes the body to retain water and bloat. Stock your refrigerator with perishable foods to eliminate much of the salt, the fat, and the added chemicals that are found in processed and canned foods. And don't forget to drink water throughout the entire day to get rid of toxins and flush out your system, keeping your body healthy and hydrated.

- Take a sauna. It's great for sweating out all of those toxins and excess fluids. It only has a temporary effect, however, and you, unlike a boxer, must keep hydrated. Boxers dehydrate until we get off the scale, then we guzzle the fluids! You've got to replace not only the water you'll sweat, but electrolytes such as sodium and potassium.

You've really made progress with this program, and to you I say, "Way to go!" The body and the success you want will be yours if you'll just remember to do a few more things.

One key to your success will be to push yourself beyond what you think you can do (without hurting yourself). Most of the time you'll find that you can accomplish so much more than you originally thought you could.

Another thing I want you to do is be good to yourself. A lot of times we don't give ourselves enough credit. Every morning, I want you to look in the mirror and tell yourself, "I love you. You are beautiful, smart, and kind. And you have a beautiful body." Repeat those words ten times every day, and watch how quickly you will start to see these qualities.

You'll begin to notice that the better you feel about yourself, the easier it is to start your workout. Talk to yourself while you are working out, saying, "I can do this. I feel light as a feather. I am fast and strong, and I can keep going as long as I want. My body will not crumble, and neither will my mind or spirit." Create your own power affirmations that make you feel great, and the results will amaze you.

Always know that you have the power to change. All of the power you need to fulfill your dreams is inside you right now. Once you let go of your old beliefs, ideas, attitudes, and habits in regard to exercise, eating, and thinking, and start using the strategies I've shared with you, you will transform your body and mind and embark on a road toward unimagined success.

9

Knockout Workout Recipes

This is the most delicious part of the book. I've included some of my favorite meals, snacks, and recipes, created by my mother, Maria Elena Socorro Rosales. Not only does she work my corner as a second (a second works beside the main coach), but she keeps me on a healthy eating plan, and this is no easy task.

My mother was born and raised in Zacatecas, Mexico, in a small town named Barrio de la Cantera. Besides being a great cook, my mother is such an inspiration to me. I wouldn't be the success I am without her. She spoke no English before coming to the United States, yet she encouraged me to graduate from college and fulfill all of my dreams.

When I was a child, I was raised on beans, rice, tortillas, and carne asada, so, needless to say, I was kind of chubby. Mom began to develop recipes for me when I first started boxing. She knew that for me to stay on weight for my fights, the Mexican food I was raised on would have to be altered. The trick was that we had to find a way for me to continue eating the foods I loved and had grown up on, but to do so in a healthier way, so that I could maintain a lean fighting weight.

I'm happy to say we managed to do this. My mother's recipes helped me reach my goal every weigh-in day. This section includes some of her unique recipes, many of which have a Latin flair. This chapter lists some Latin dishes that typically are high-carb and high-fat, but these alternative versions are healthier, leaner, and just as tasty.

Breakfast

Protein-Filled Breakfast of Champions

SERVES 1

½ scoop protein powder

8 ounces fat-free yogurt

1 teaspoon wheat germ*

1 tablespoon natural peanut butter

4 ounces cold orange juice

4 ounces cold water

Combine all of the ingredients in a blender and blend on high speed for 30 to 40 seconds.

Vitamin C Breakfast

SERVES 1

1 cup grapefruit juice

½ scoop soy protein

1 tablespoon diet sugar (Sweet 'n' Low, Splenda, Equal, or other)

1 teaspoon wheat germ

crushed ice

Combine the first four ingredients in a blender, add the crushed ice to taste, and blend on high speed for 30 to 40 seconds.

Wheat germ is a good source of vitamin E and folic acid.

If you're hungry for a good old-fashioned hot dog, try the low-fat and nonfat turkey or chicken franks. I know, you're thinking a hot dog should be beef or pork, but take a good look at the label next time you're in the store. Some of those regular hot dogs can have upward of 15 grams of fat *per* hot dog. Yikes!

Energy Breakfast
SERVES 1

1 cup fat-free milk
1/2 scoop protein powder
1 teaspoon wheat germ

1 cup strawberries
crushed ice

In a blender, combine the first four ingredients. Add the crushed ice to taste, and blend.

Pancakes with Oatmeal and Blueberries
SERVES 2

1 1/2 cups oatmeal, dry, the
   quick-cooking kind
2 eggs
2 cups fat-free milk

3 teaspoons olive oil
1 teaspoon strawberry extract
   (if desired)
1 cup blueberries

In a mixing bowl, combine all of the ingredients except the berries to form a batter. Then add the blueberries. Heat 1 teaspoon of oil at a time in a nonstick pan. Pour the batter into the pan to make 6 small or 4 medium-size pancakes.

Quick Blueberry Breakfast
Serves 1

1 cup cold fat-free milk
1/2 cup blueberries

1/2 scoop soy protein

Combine all of the ingredients in a blender and blend to taste.

Quick Breakfast with Cottage Cheese and Blueberries
SERVES 2

1 cup cottage cheese
1 scoop protein powder
1 cup sliced strawberries

1 cup blueberries
12 sliced almonds
2 drops banana extract

In a mixing bowl, combine all of the ingredients and blend.

Protein-Packed Oatmeal
SERVES 1

1 cup dry "old-fashioned"
   slow-cooking oats
2 cups water

3 tablespoons protein powder
cinnamon (to taste)
1 tablespoon sliced almonds

Cook the oatmeal in the water according to the package directions. Remove it from the heat. Stir in the protein powder, cinnamon, and almonds. Substitute 1 cup of nonfat milk or 2 egg whites for 1 tablespoon of protein powder. If you are using 1 cup nonfat milk, reduce the water to 1 cup.

Scrambled Eggs
Serves 1

$^1/_3$ teaspoon olive oil
4 egg whites
1 ounce nonfat cheese, cut
   in small cubes

3 tablespoons nonfat milk
1 piece whole-grain bread
$^1/_2$ teaspoon natural peanut butter

Coat a nonstick pan with the olive oil. In a bowl, beat the eggs with the nonfat cheese. Add the nonfat milk to the eggs, then scramble. Toast the bread and spread the peanut butter on it. Drink coffee, milk, or juice, or eat $^1/_2$ of an apple instead of drinking juice.

Omelette à la Mexicana
Serves 1

2 teaspoons olive oil
1 tablespoon onion, minced
1 garlic clove, minced, add to taste
1/2 cup cooked pinto beans, or
    your choice
1 tablespoon red bell pepper, diced
1/2 cup mushrooms, minced

1 whole egg
2 egg whites
black pepper, to taste
hot sauce, to taste
turmeric, to taste
1/2 teaspoon chili powder, or to taste
nonfat cheese for sprinkling, to taste

In a nonstick pan, heat 1 teaspoon of oil. Cook the onion, garlic, beans, red pepper, and mushrooms until tender. In a mixing bowl, whip together the whole egg, egg whites, black pepper, hot sauce, turmeric, and chili powder. In a second nonstick pan, heat 1 teaspoon of oil, add the egg mixture, and cook until set and an omelet is formed. Fill the omelet with the vegetable mixture and fold it over, sprinkle it with nonfat cheese, and serve.

Lunch or Dinner

Rice with Vegetables
Serves 2

2 cups washed rice (brown or white)
3 tablespoons olive oil
2 cups water
1/2 cup onions, sliced
1 cup celery, sliced

1/2 cup cilantro, chopped
1 red pepper, sliced
2 small green onions, chopped
1/4 cup lemon juice
garlic, salt, and pepper to taste

Place the rice in a nonstick pan and lightly brown it. Add the olive oil and 1/2 cup of onions and cover this with water. When the rice is amost cooked, add the celery, cilantro, red pepper, green onions, lemon, garlic, salt, and pepper, the last 3 items to taste. Cook the rice al dente or to taste. Add more (hot) water if it's needed. Serve the rice with fish, salmon, chicken, or any meat of your choice.

Many people are confused when they hear they should be eating a certain number of servings of this or that food from a certain food group. Do you know how big a serving is? Here's an easy way to remember: $1/2$ to 1 cup of cooked or raw vegetables is one serving, $1/2$ cup of vegetable or fruit juice is one serving, and one medium-size piece of fruit is also one serving. And what about fish, fowl, or meat portion sizes? Aim for a serving (about 3 to 4 ounces) that's about the size of a computer mouse or a folded wallet.

Chickpea Salad

Serves 1

1 chicken breast, cooked, sliced

$1/2$ cup chickpeas, cooked

$1/2$ teaspoon yellow lemon zest, grated

1 teaspoon olive oil

1 green onion, sliced (optional)

6 green olives

salt and pepper to taste

2 tomato slices

1 slice avocado

In a mixing bowl, combine the chicken, chickpeas, lemon zest, olive oil, green onion (if using), green olives, and salt and pepper (to taste). Use lemon or another dressing of your choice. Decorate the salad with tomato and avocado slices.

Taco Salad

Serves 1

1 tablespoon olive oil

6 ounces diet ground beef
   (less than 10 percent fat)

1 green onion, sliced

3 tablespoons low-sodium taco
   seasoning mix

2 cups romaine lettuce

$1/4$ avocado, sliced

1 medium red tomato, sliced

1 ounce fat-free cheddar cheese

3 tablespoons salsa, if desired

In a nonstick pan, heat the oil, ground beef, green onion, and taco seasoning, and cook until the meat is done. In a medium bowl, toss the lettuce, then top it with the ground beef mixture, avocado, tomato, cheese, and salsa to taste.

Tuna-Stuffed Tomato
Serves 2

4 ounces tuna, packed in water
2 large firm red tomatoes
3 tablespoons mayonnaise

1 stalk celery, diced
salt and pepper, to taste

Drain the excess water from the tuna. In a bowl, mix the tuna, mayonnaise, celery, and seasonings. Cut the tomatoes in halves, scoop out the pulp, and set them aside. If the tuna mixture is dry, add some of the tomato pulp to make it moist, and fill the tomato shells with the tuna.

Chicken with Mushrooms
Serves 1

3 ounces chicken, skinless, roasted, sliced
1 cup mushrooms
1 cup romaine lettuce

2 slices red tomato
6 green olives
lemon juice or vinegar

In a mixing bowl, combine all of the ingredients. Use the lemon juice or vinegar for a dressing.

Quick Enchiladas
Serves 4

1 (2-ounce) can green chiles
2 tablespoons olive oil
1 clove garlic, minced
2 green onions, chopped
2 tomatoes, chopped
salt to taste
pinch dry oregano

$1/2$ cup water
2 chicken breasts, cooked and
   chopped
8 ounces mozzarella cheese
$1/2$ cup light sour cream
8 tortillas

Drain the chiles, rinse the seeds off, and chop. Heat the oil in a nonstick pan. Sauté the chiles, garlic, and onions. Add the tomatoes and stir in the salt, oregano, and water. Simmer this uncovered until it is slightly thickened. Heat the oven to 350 degrees Fahrenheit. Combine the chicken with $1/2$ of the cheese and sour cream, spread this mixture on the tortillas, and roll them up. Place them in a shallow pan. Spread the rest of the cheese over them, and cook for 20 minutes or until hot and bubbling.

Quick Turkey

Serves 1

2½ cups broccoli, steamed

4 ounces turkey breast, skinless

1 slice canned cranberry sauce

2 small slices avocado

Place the broccoli and turkey on a plate. Decorate them with the cranberry sauce and avocado slices. Serve this for lunch or a snack.

Fish Delight

Serves 1

olive oil cooking spray

4½ ounces fish fillet (flounder)

chopped onion, to taste

salt and pepper, to taste

1 teaspoon lemon juice

1 tablespoon Parmesan cheese

½ tomato, sliced

6 green olives

Spray a piece of aluminum foil with the olive oil cooking spray. Place the fish fillet in the center of the foil, along with the onion, salt and pepper, lemon juice, and cheese. Add the tomatoes and olives, or save them for a garnish after the fish has cooked. Fold the foil over the fish, leaving a pocket of air around the fish. Seal the sides and the middle to prevent the juice from leaking. Bake it in a 425-degree oven for 18 minutes. Serve the fish with a spinach or romaine lettuce salad, along with an orange for dessert.

Cheeseburger Delight

Serves 1

4½ ounces lean hamburger

1 slice nonfat or reduced-fat cheese

1 slice whole-grain bread

2 slices tomato

1 romaine lettuce leaf

1 slice onion (optional)

salt and pepper, to taste

Broil the hamburger in a 500-degree Fahrenheit oven (with the degree of doneness to your taste). Place the cheese on top of the hamburger and return it to the oven for a few seconds until the cheese melts. Serve the burger on whole-grain bread, topped with tomatoes, lettuce, and onion (optional). Add the salt and pepper to taste. Serve it with ½ apple and 6 raw almonds for dessert.

Grilled or Steamed Chicken
Serves 1

1 chicken breast, skinless
salt and pepper, to taste
2 lemon slices

2 onion slices, if desired
1 tablespoon olive oil

Steam the chicken (you may also grill it, if you prefer). Season it with salt and pepper. Add the lemon and onion slices or save as a garnish after the chicken is cooked. If you are grilling, coat the chicken with the olive oil. Serve the meal with 1 cup of berries for dessert (blueberries, strawberries, or boysenberries).

Chicken with Vegetables
Serves 4

1 cup celery, sliced
2 basil leaves
$1/2$ tablespoon olive oil
6 slices red bell pepper
6 slices yellow bell pepper
7-ounce can tomato salsa
$1/2$ cup chicken broth
   (fat-free)
salt and pepper, to taste
garlic, minced, to taste

2 chicken breasts, cooked and
   sliced into 4 equal-size pieces
8 green or black olives
8 slices cucumber
8 slices red tomato
1 medium avocado, quartered
1 tablespoon refried beans
low-fat cheese, grated (sprinkle on
   to taste)
wheat-flour tortillas

Place the celery and basil leaves in a cooking pan over medium heat. Add the olive oil and the green and red bell peppers. Add the 7-ounce can of salsa. Add the chicken broth. Bring it to a boil. Add the salt, pepper, and garlic to taste. Add the chicken. Cook it until the chicken is hot, then remove the pan from the stove. Decorate the dish with the olives, cucumber, tomato, avocado, and refried beans. Sprinkle it with low-fat cheese. Serve one tortilla per person.

Tostadas with Turkey
Serves 1

4 ounces lean turkey, ground
1 teaspoon olive oil
1/2 tablespoon onions, minced, or to taste
1 tablespoon green pepper, minced
1 tablespoon red pepper, minced
1/2 teaspoon chili powder
black pepper to taste

oregano to taste
1/2 cup cooked pinto beans
  or your choice
1/2 cup tomato sauce
2 corn tostadas
sprinkling of nonfat cheese
1/2 fresh tomato, sliced

Brown the meat in the olive oil with the onions, green and red peppers, and spices, and stir often. Add the cooked beans and the tomato sauce and cook, stirring occasionally, for 5 minutes or until the meat and vegetables are cooked. Serve this over 2 corn tostadas. Top them with the cheese and tomatoes.

Mexican Beef Fajitas for Two
Serves 2

1 2/3 cup olive oil
10 ounces lean beef (in small slices)
1/2 tablespoon chili powder
1/2 cup salsa

4 corn tortillas

1 cup tomato, diced fine
1 tablespoon onion, minced
1/2 teaspoon garlic, minced
9 black olives, diced

Beans
1 cup cooked pinto beans, kidney
  beans, or black beans, rinsed

1/2 cup salsa
1 slice fat-free cheese

BEEF INSTRUCTIONS
In a nonstick sauté pan, add the olive oil, and when it's hot, add the beef, chili powder, 1/2 cup of salsa, diced tomato, onion, garlic, and olives, and cook. Spoon the mixture onto the tortillas.

BEANS INSTRUCTIONS
Warm the beans and add 1/2 cup salsa, cover this with cheese, and serve with the tortillas.

Chicken Quesadilla Marraton

Serves 2

1 teaspoon olive oil

2 flour tortillas

2 ounces nonfat cheese

1 chicken breast, cooked and diced

4 tablespoons guacamole

2 tablespoons cilantro, chopped

$1/2$ cup salsa

In a large warm nonstick pan, pour in $1/2$ of the olive oil and spread it over the pan. Place a tortilla in the pan and cover $1/2$ of the tortilla with $1/2$ of the cheese and $1/2$ of the chicken. Flip the empty $1/2$ of the tortilla over to make a soft taco. Place it on a plate. Repeat the same step with the next tortilla. Once both tortillas are folded, place them back in the pan over medium heat for a minute or until the cheese starts to melt. Flip both tortillas to the other side and cook them for another minute or until the cheese is melted. Place them on a plate and spread $1/2$ of the guacamole over each, sprinkle on the cilantro, and add salsa to taste.

Lemon Chicken

Serves 4

$2^1/2$ tablespoons extra-virgin olive oil

4 chicken breasts, boneless and skinless

salt and pepper, to taste

4 bay leaves

1 tablespoon garlic, chopped

2 tablespoons scallions, sliced

1 red bell pepper, sliced

1 teaspoon dry basil

1 teaspoon dry oregano

2 tablespoons lemon juice

1 lemon, sliced

Heat the oven to 375 degrees Fahrenheit. Coat a large nonstick pan with $1/2$ tablespoon of the olive oil. Season the chicken with the salt and pepper. Place the chicken breasts in a single layer with the bay leaves in between the 4 pieces. In a mixing bowl, blend the oil, garlic, scallions, bell pepper, basil, oregano, and lemon juice. Cover the chicken with the mixture. Place the lemon slices over the mixture. Bake it for 15 minutes. Remove the lemon slices to the side of the chicken. Turn the breasts once. Cook them 5 minutes longer or until they're fully cooked. Remove the bay leaves and lemon slices before serving.

Side Dishes

Potato Mex

Serves 2 to 4

1½ pounds red potatoes, sliced
2 tablespoons olive oil
1 tablespoon dry rosemary
2 tablespoons scallions, sliced
1 tomato, chopped

garlic, minced, to taste
salt and pepper, to taste
Parmesan cheese, to taste
1 tablespoon parsley, chopped

Heat the oven to 450 degrees Fahrenheit. Place all of the ingredients except the cheese and parsley in a roasting pan and cover them with foil. Cook the potatoes for 25 minutes. Remove the foil and stir. Sprinkle the potatoes with the Parmesan cheese and fresh parsley. Cook them for an additional 15 to 20 minutes.

Almond Spinach

Serves 4

1 tablespoon olive oil
1 tablespoon garlic, chopped
1 tablespoon raw almonds, sliced

1 pound spinach, raw
salt and pepper, to taste

In a nonstick pan, add the olive oil and garlic over medium heat. Sauté the garlic to a light golden color. Add the almonds and spinach, and cook until the spinach is wilted. Add the salt and pepper to taste.

DID YOU KNOW THAT... A 4-ounce serving of french fries has almost three times the calories and more than 10 times the waist-expanding amount of fat when compared to a 4-ounce baked potato. If you love french fries (and who doesn't), then try baking them instead of frying. It's a great taste with minimal fat.

Snacks and Desserts

Cottage Cheese Dessert

Serves 1

1/2 cup cottage cheese
1 tablespoon wheat germ
1 tablespoon sliced almonds

artificial or regular sugar, to taste
1/2 cup sliced strawberries

In a mixing bowl, mix the cottage cheese, wheat germ, and almonds. Add the sweetener or sugar. Spoon the mixture into a dessert bowl or a sherbet cup and top with the strawberries.

Quick Energizer

Serves 1

1 cup fat-free milk
1/2 banana
1 cup strawberries

1/2 scoop protein powder
crushed ice

Combine the first four ingredients in a blender. Add the crushed ice to taste and blend.

INDEX